H. J. Deeg H.-G. Klingemann G. L. Phillips

A Guide to Bone Marrow Transplantation

Springer-Verlag
Berlin Heidelberg New York
London Paris Tokyo

Hans Joachim Deeg, M.D.

Vincent T. Lombardi Cancer Research Center
Georgetown University Medical Center
3800 Reservoir Road, N.W.
Washington, D.C. 20007, USA

Hans-Georg Klingemann, M.D.

Leukemia/Bone Marrow Transplant Program of B.C.
University of British Columbia
910 West 10th Avenue
Vancouver, B.C., Canada

Gordon L. Phillips, M.D.

Leukemia/Bone Marrow Transplant Program of B.C.
University of British Columbia
910 West 10th Avenue
Vancouver, B.C., Canada

ISBN-13:978-3-642-97079-5 e-ISBN-13:978-3-642-97077-1
DOI: 10.1007/978-3-642-97077-1

Softcover reprint of the hardcover 1st edition 1988

2127/3140/543210

Preface

In the late 1940s investigators observed that mice given supralethal doses of total body irradiation were protected by infusion of viable spleen or marrow cells following irradiation, and that this was accomplished by hemopoietic reconstitution with donor cells as proven using genetic markers. If a similar approach could be applied to humans, it should be possible to treat leukemia patients with any dose of chemoradiotherapy as far as nonmarrow toxicity permitted, and then rescue them by marrow transplantation. Early clinical attempts were generally unsuccessful, mostly due to a lack of knowledge of histocompatibility antigens and appropriate supportive care. These areas developed rather quickly during the 1960s, and for almost two decades now clinical marrow transplantation has been carried out with increasing success. After initially using only bone marrow from HLA indentical siblings, the field has expanded rapidly to incorporate HLA nonidentical related donors, and recently even marrow from unrelated volunteer donors. Furthermore, since for numerous patients who otherwise could benefit from transplantation a donor cannot be identified, there has been a growing interest in using the patient's own (autologous) bone marrow.

Our understanding of the principles of transplantation and our knowledge of the potential risks and benefits have quickly grown. At times it is difficult, however, to decide what is the best option for a given patient. This problem is further accentuated by the fact that the nontransplant management of the patients under consideration (e.g., patients with severe aplastic anemia, acute or chronic leukemia, lymphomas) has improved concurrently. Rather than being used in a complementary fashion, they have often been presented as competing options. Therefore, we felt that there was a need for a text that would address these issues. Conceivably, if all treatment options including bone marrow transplantation are included in treatment planning early after a patient's diagnosis is established, they can be applied more intelligently, hopefully with reduced toxicity, and hence at less risk for the patient. Consequently long-term results should improve. From a psychological point of view this may also allow a patient more time to weigh the various options and adjust to potential problems.

Although this book is directed primarily at internists and pediatricians, in particular hematologists and oncologists treating patients who might benefit bone marrow transplantation, we believe that it will also be of interest to other physicians, students and physicians in training, nurses, technologists involved in marrow transplantations, patients, and possibly those involved in insurance questions and other administrative aspects.

Our aim was to present each chapter and section in this book as a closed entity. Of necessity this has led to some overlap and duplication of sections of the discussion which appear to be pertinent in more than one place. We believe this may actually be an advantage since the readers will find any topic of interest under one heading rather than having to go through the entire book.

We are indebted to our teachers who introduced us to the exciting field of bone marrow transplantation, to our patients who gave us the gratifying experience of success, and to our colleagues and students who continue to challenge our views. We would like to thank our secretaries for their never-fatiguing support during the preparation of the manuscript, and the staff of Springer-Verlag, especially Dr. J. Wieczorek, for their responsiveness to our requests and the ability to accommodate last-minute modifications. We hope that we have not neglected any of our other duties during the preparation of the manuscript, but if we have done so we hope that the benefits of this book will allow us to make good for it.

H. Joachim Deeg
Hans-Georg Klingemann
Gordon L. Phillips

Contents

I. Introduction

The goal of any cancer therapy is to eradicate malignant cells. The extent of cell kill is dependent upon the sensitivity of the cells and the dose of chemo- or radiotherapy administered. For many treatment modalities the dose limiting factor is myelosuppression. Therefore, it is often impossible to give the maximum desired dose since patients would succumb to bone marrow aplasia and associated complications such as hemorrhage and infection.

Attempts at the therapeutic use of bone marrow for the treatment of various forms of anemia or leukemia were made as early as 1891. A true transplant attempt, for severe aplastic anemia, was first reported in 1939. All these experiments antedated, of course, the recognition of histocompatibility antigens in man and were carried out without immunosuppressive or cytotoxic treatment of the patient. In retrospect, therefore, it is not surprising that none of these attempts were successful.

In the late 1940's several investigators began to experiment with total body irradiation (TBI) in animal models. These workers distinguished three dose-dependent irradiation syndromes: the marrow syndrome (marrow aplasia with infection and hermorrhage) at doses of 5 to 7 Gy, the intestinal syndrome (bowel damage with fluid and electrolyte loss) at 12 to 100 Gy, and a central nervous system (CNS) syndrome (CNS damage with seizures and uncontrolled sympathetic and parasympathetic functions) at doses $>$ 100 Gy. These workers also noted that mice irradiated with doses higher than those leading to marrow aplasia, but lower than those resulting in a lethal intestinal syndrome would survive if the spleen was shielded, or alternatively, if spleen or spleen cells were transplanted to the irradiated mouse after TBI. Subsequently it was proven that hemopoietic and lymphopoietic recovery in these animals was not due to endogenous recovery of autologous cells, possibly stimulated by a humoral factor, but rather due to engraftment of transplanted stem cells. Similar results could be achieved by using modalities other than TBI, such as cytotoxic drugs, to prepare the recipient for engraftment. Recipients carrying a lymphohemopoietic system derived from a different individual are called "chimeras".

It was in these animal models that most of the problems subsequently encountered in clinical transplantation were first recognized. Aside from toxicity related to the conditioning regimen problems included hemorrhage, infection, fluid and electrolyte imbalance, and most importantly "secondary disease", subsequently called graft-vs-host disease (GVHD). GVHD is a syndrome observed in marrow transplant recipients given marrow from donors other than genotypically identical, monozygotic (syngeneic) twins. This reaction is initiated by donor T lymphocytes which recognize, in the recipient, histocompatibility antigens (major or minor) that differ from those present in the donor. This recognition leads to a destructive process originally directed at lymphohemopoietic cells of the recipient. Associated with this reaction are clinical manifestations in the host (patient), classically described in skin, liver, and intestinal tract, but also recognized in other tissues such as the conjunctivae. GVHD can be associated with substantial morbidity and mortality, due either directly to GVHD or to associated complications, especially infections. GVHD also retards the already slow post grafting immune recovery seen in marrow transplant recipients. Consequently, efforts have been directed at preventing GVHD either by treating transplant patients with immunosuppressive agents such as methotrexate, cyclophosphamide and cyclosporine after transplantation or by removing donor T-lymphocytes from the marrow before infusion into the recipient. These approaches have improved overall transplant results, but have not been uniformly successful. In particular, the elimination of T-lymphocytes from donor marrow in vitro has resulted in a new problem, i.e. failure to achieve sustained engraftment even in HLA identical transplant recipients.

The present text is meant to serve as a general guide to bone marrow transplantation. It includes considerations from the time of diagnosis, goes through the process of donor selection, the acutal transplant procedure, acute and chronic transplant-related problems, and long term observations. We did not intend this book to teach physicians how to carry out marrow transplants. Rather, this text should help physicians to decide who among their patients might benefit from transplantation, when it should ideally be carried out, and what studies should be obtained to provide a basis for discussion with and referral to a marrow transplant center. It should also help physicians with the management of potential problems that might be expected post transplant after the patient returns home.

Several questions such as histocompatibility typing, timing of transplantation, toxicity in individual organs are discussed in more than one place. Although this has resulted in some unavoidable overlap, it also allows the readers to find relevant information in the context of various questions they may be interested in.

References

van Bekkum DW, De Vries MJ (1967) Radiation Chimeras, Logos Press Ltd., London

Blume KG, Petz LD (1983) Clinical Bone Marrow Transplantation. Churchill Livingston, New York

Bortin MM, Rimm AA (1986) Increasing utilization of bone marrow transplantation. Transplantation 42: 229

O'Reilly RJ (1983) Allogeneic bone marrow transplantation: current status and future directions. Blood 62: 941

Philip T, Armitage JO, Spitzer G, Chauvin F, Jagannath S, Cahn J-Y, Colombat P, Goldstone AH, Gorin NC, Flesh M, Laporte J-P, Maraninchi D, Pico J, Bosly A, Anderson C, shots R, Biron P, Cabanillas F, Dicke K (1987) High-dose therapy and autologous bone marrow

transplantation after failure of conventional chemotherapy in adults with intermediate-grade or high-grade non-Hodgkin's lymphoma. N Eng J Med 316: 1493
Santos GW (1983) History of bone marrow transplantation. Clinics in Hematol 12: 611
Storb R, Thomas ED (1983) Allogeneic bone-marrow transplantation. Immunol Rev 71: 77
Thomas ED, Storb R, Clift RA, Fefer A, Johnson FL, Neiman PE, Lerner KG, Glucksberg H, Buckner CD (1975) Bone-marrow transplantation (Parts I & 2) New Eng J Med 17: 832; 895

II. Pre-Transplant Considerations

1. How Should Marrow Transplantation be Approached?

Marrow transplantation is no longer a last desperate effort aimed only at salvaging patients with far advanced disease. Marrow transplantation in 1988 is a well established modality, which may acutally represent the treatment of choice for a given patient, and hence, should be part of treatment planning early in the patient's course. This can be a demanding task, but the approach is generally rewarding both for physicians and patients. There must be no misunderstanding: marrow transplantation is a complex and expensive therapy. Results depend upon factors such as disease stage, patient age, histocompatibility, possibly donor age, and the patient's overall medical condition. Some transplants, especially autologous, are still considered experimental and may not be covered by health insurance. Early recognition and discussion of potential problems may allow for them to be resolved, may direct therapeutic efforts in different directions, or may provide time needed to assure financing.

Table 1 lists diagnoses for which marrow transplantation has been carried out. While this list may be incomplete, since indications are constantly expanding, it should be helpful in determining which patients are likely to be transplant candidates.

Table 1. Diseases Treated With Marrow Transplantation

Malignant	Nonmalignant	
	Acquired	Congenital
Acute Nonlymphoblastic Leukemia	Aplastic anemia	Immunodeficiencies
Acute Lymphoblastic Leukemia	Paroxysmal nocturnal hemoglobinuria	Hematologic defects
		Bone defects
Chronic Myelogenous Leukemia	Myelofibrosis	Mucopolysaccharidoses
		Mucolipidoses
Non-Hodgkin's Lymphoma		Other lysosomal diseases
Hodgkin's Disease		
Multiple Myeloma		
Preleukemia		
Hairy Cell Leukemia		
Selected solid tumors		

The diagnosis of illness often generates a feeling of helplessness, and in the case of malignancy or a non-malignant but frequently fatal disorder evokes the impression of being doomed. There is despair, anger, and revolt against accepting such a sentence. A detailed discussion of options and prognosis is frequently helpful. Such a discussion is best led by someone expert in the field. In fact, patients will often inquire about whom they could talk to, or where they could go to receive the best available counseling and treatment. If a patient is already being treated at an established transplant center, none of these questions may pose a problem. However, a different approach may have to be taken if the patient is undergoing treatment at a medical center where transplantation is not carried out. Thus, a good coordinating effort between patient, physician, and transplant center is necessary.

Treatment Planning

As soon as a patient has been identified as one who might benefit from marrow transplantation, the transplant option should be incorporated in the overall therapeutic plan. A most important aspect is the timing of transplantation. This question is discussed in detail below (II.2.). The major problem in this context is that both transplant and non-transplant approaches and respective results change over time. For example, as long term disease free survival in children with acute lymphoblastic leukemia (ALL) has improved over the years, the use of marrow transplantation in first remission ALL has frequently been questioned. It is necessary to constantly re-evaluate and reassess the available therapeutic modalities. As new chemotherapeutic agents are found effective in treating various leukemias, such agents will be incorporated in the preparative regimens for marrow transplantation. Consequently both transplant and non-transplant results may improve. Toxicity associated with marrow transplantation can be severe. The addition of new agents either to the non-transplant regimen, or to the transplant conditioning regimen might add further toxicity and may affect transplant related complications and quality of long term survival. Numerous such interactions between different agents, not observed previously, have recently been reported. Similarly, various risk factors have been recognized in patients with nonmalignant disease such as aplastic anemia which have also influenced the timing of marrow transplantation.

Congenital Disorders. One of the classic indications for marrow transplantation is severe combined immunodeficiency (SCID). Since these children rarely live longer than one year, there is agreement that marrow transplantation must be carried out early. HLA typing of the affected child, siblings, and parents should be obtained expeditiously to determine if an HLA identical donor not affected by the disease is available. However, even if this is not the case, plans for transplantation should be pursued further. Recent developments of T cell depletion of the donor marrow (see below) have allowed for successful transplantation even from a haploidentical parent. Since immunosuppression of the recipient in preparation for transplantation is generally not necessary (due to the underlying immunodeficiency state) there need be no concern in regards to cumulative toxicity of various treatments that might be given prior to transplantation. In some children fetal liver cell transplantation has been attempted and successful outcome has been reported by several teams.

There are additional congenital immunodeficiencies which can be approached similarly. These diseases include the bare lymphocyte syndrome, ionophor responsive combined immunodeficiency, combined immunodeficiency with a capping abnormality, and nucleoside phosphorylase deficiency.

Most important in all these patients is the prevention of infections prior to transplantation at any cost, since the presence of infections will substantially increase the risk of dying from complications after transplantation. As soon as a diagnosis of immunodeficiency is established, or only suspected, an experienced transplant center should be contacted for further management of the patient, and presumably the patient should be referred there for evaluation.

There are other congenital disorders of immunodeficiency which usually allow for a somewhat longer survival of the affected individual. These include the Wiskott-Aldrich syndrome, chronic granulomatous disease, ataxia-telangiectasia, cartilage-hair hypoplasia, and others listed in Table 2. These diagnoses may allow for more time to observe the patient, evaluate siblings (if available) and parents before a decision for transplantation is made. In contrast to patients with combined immunodeficiencies, these patients generally require immunosuppressive conditioning (by drugs or irradiation or a combination of both) to achieve sustained engraftment even with HLA identical bone marrow. Hence, pretransplant treatment in the form of antithymocyte globulin and blood product transfusions may well have an effect on the toxicity associated with conditioning for marrow transplantation.

Table 2. Congenital Disorders Treated by Marrow Transplantation

Immunodeficiencies	Mucopolysaccharidoses
– Severe Combined Immunodeficiency	– Hurler Syndrome
– Chronic Mucocutaneous Candidiasis	– Hunter Syndrome
	– Maroteaux-Lamy Syndrome
– Others	– Others
Hematologic Defects	Mucolipidoses
	– Metachromatic Leukodystrophy
– Wiscott-Aldrich Syndrome	– Other Lipidoses
– Fanconi's Anemia	– Adrenoleukodystrophy
– Blackfan-Diamond Anemia	Other Lysosomal Diseases
– Thalassemia	– Lesch-Nyhan Syndrome
– Sickel Cell Disease	
– Glanzman Thrombasthenia	– Type IIa Glycogen Storage Disease
– Gaucher Disease	
– Chronic Granulomatous Disease	
– Congenital Neutropenia	
– Chediak Higashi Syndrome	
Osteopetrosis	

Recently metabolic storage diseases have also been treated successfully by marrow transplantation. Some of these are listed in Table 2. The number of patients transplanted to date is limited, but a good proportion of these still survive. It is of note that engraftment of allogeneic marrow is usually not a problem, although GVHD has developed in a number of patients. It appears, therefore, that transfusions given prior to transplantation may not have a negative effect on engraftment, and that engraftment can be achieved easily. Nevertheless, a transplant center should be contacted as soon as the diagnosis has been established.

In patients with Fanconi's anemia, transplants have generally been carried out when severe marrow hypoplasia and pancytopenia develop. Since in these patients toxicity associated with transplantation has often been more severe than in patients with other diagnoses (e.g. severe aplastic anemia), conditioning regimens have been modified accordingly. Again, it is of note that failure of engraftment is usually not a problem. However, one should consider that patients with Franconi's anemia are at a significant risk of developing secondary malignancies including preleukemia and leukemia even if they do not develop marrow hypoplasia. Although these diseases have also been treated successfully by marrow transplantation, it might be preferable to treat the patient earlier, at a time when there is no evidence of malignant transformation. Transfusion-induced sensitization prior to marrow transplantation has not been a problem.

A very large target group for marrow transplantation are patients with thalassemia major. Both patients and physicians sense the decision about marrow transplantation as a dilemma (see II.2. below). It is helpful to consult a transplant physician who has experience with this disease early in the patient's course. It also seems prudent to recommend judicious transfusion support and to make efforts to avoid sensitization. These considerations are important since both the nature of the disease, with a "turned-on" hypercellular marrow, and the sensitization status of the patient may have a negative impact on marrow engraftment. Although we are not dealing with a malignant disease, the abnormal hemopoietic stem cells apparently have a growth advantage. They are at times difficult to eradicate and thalassemia can recur after transplantation.

Severe Aplastic Anemia. Aplastic anemia is a nonmalignant but often lethal disease. At the present time there are two major modalities of treatment:

a) immunosuppresion, usually in the form of antihymocyte globulin, (a limited number of patients has also been treated with cyclosporine or monoclonal antibodies), and
b) bone marrow transplantation.

Although some centers have reported very encouraging results with immunosuppression, in general survival appears to be superior with marrow transplantation. Furthermore, patients usually become hemopoietically normal after transplant, but not after immunosuppression. Due to the nature of the disease, of course, autologous transplantation is not an option and therefore a healthy allogeneic, or in rare instances, syngeneic donor must be available.

Severe aplastic anemia is not one single entity, but probably comprises a spectrum of syndromes. Clinically these are quite similar, but etiologically they may differ significantly. Common to all patients with aplastic anemia, however, has been a very high probability of marrow graft rejection, ranging from 30–60% in early studies. Most analyses have indicated that rejection was due to the fact that patients had been sensitized by transfusions before marrow transplant. For this reason it is desirable to carry out transplants in untransfused patients. Indeed, subsequent studies using this approach were quite rewarding. Untransfused patients were significantly less likely to reject the marrow graft than transfused patients. This implies that any physician diagnosing a patients with severe aplastic anemia should, whenever possible, avoid transfusions and obtain HLA typing expeditiously so that the patient can be referred to a transplant center for transplantation while still untransfused. This is certainly true for patients up to approximately 45 years of age. Since the older age population has a substantially higher risk of transplant-associated complications, it may be worthwhile to consider immunosuppressive therapy as the first line approach. Only if this fails would one then consider a marrow transplant if a suitable donor is available (see II.2 below).

Most transplants in patients with aplastic anemia have been from HLA identical sibling donors since the incidence of rejection is higher with histoincompatible donors. However, it is clear now that the lack of an HLA identical sibling per se is not reason enough *not* to pursue the possibility of marrow transplantation. Several transplants from HLA matched unrelated volunteer donors have been reported, and such a search should be initiated, particularly if the patient's HLA type represents a common HLA phenotype in a given population (Table 3). Further, several transplants have been carried out from donors, usually blood relatives, who were not completely HLA identical, but differed for a least one HLA antigen. This usually required more severe immunosuppression of the patient, generally in the form of TBI, but successful engraftment and long term survival have been reported.

In any event an early consultation with a transplant center should be obtained. Frequently, the recommendation by the experts will be that not only older patients (see above), but also younger patients, who do not have a complete match, should be given immunosuppression as initial therapy before marrow transplan-

Table 3. Common HLA-A, B Haplotypes and B/DR Associations in Caucasians[a)]

HLA – A, B	B, DR Linkage[b)]
A1, B8	B8, DR3
A3, B7	B7, DR2
A2, Bw62	B62, DR4
A2, Bw60	Bw60, DR4
A3, Bw35	Bw35, DR1 (DR5)
A29, Bw44	Bw44, DR7 (DR4)
A1, Bw57	Bw57, DR7
A25, B18	B18, DR5 (DR3)

a) listed in order of decreasing frequency
b) most frequent (second most frequent) associated DR allele

tation is attempted. However, non-response to this management means a prolonged period of marrow hypoplasia with the associated risk of infection and hemorrhage. Transplant results in this setting, i.e. after preceding immunosuppression may be inferior to those obtained in patients in whom transplantation is used as a first line approach. Although there is no agreement as to how long after ATG therapy a response can occur, generally a patient will not "respond" to this management if there has been no improvement within 2–3 months of treatment.

What has been said for severe aplastic anemia in general also applies to paroxysmal nocturnal hemoglobinuria, once the patient develops failure of one or more cell lines.

Acute Nonlymphpoblastic Leukemia (ANL). Very aggressive and effective combination chemotherapy usually involving the use of cytosine arabinoside and daunorubicin has resulted in complete remissions in 70–80% of pediatric and adult patients. Furthermore, it has been claimed by several groups that without marrow transplantation, i.e. with chemotherapy alone, as many as 50% of patients, especially in the pediatric age group, may remain in complete, and eventually unmaintained remission. Most studies in adults suggest that about 25% of patients may remain in remission after chemotherapy only.

In the early days of marrow transplantation, all transplants were carried out in patients with far advanced, usually chemotherapy resistant acute leukemia. Encouraged by results in these endstage patients several transplant teams began in the mid 70s' to transplant patients earlier in their course, and even in first remission. Marrow transplant studies from a number of centers around the world indicate that the best results with marrow transplantation are obtained if the transplant is carried out with the patient in first chemotherapy induced remission (see II.2.). This approach has resulted in long term relapse-free survival of approximately 50–60%. However, 30% of transplanted patients still succumb to recurrent leukemia. What is the best approach at the present time? Obviously all patients require remission-induction chemotherapy. If remission is achieved, HLA typing of parents, siblings, and possibly children, should be obtained. A transplant center should be contacted. If an HLA identical sibling is available, and the patient is not more than 45 years of age, the patient should be referred for bone marrow transplantation. If the patient is older, the recommendation might be to observe the patient. Recent data analyses, particularly by the Seattle team, suggest that the relapse rate of patients transplanted for ANL in eraly relapse may not be significantly higher than the relapse rate observed after transplantation in first remission. These analyses were carried out in a retrospective fashion. If indeed this is the case, one might argue that one should induce patients into remission and observe without transplant. If relapse occurs, transplantation should be carried out expeditiously. Relapse free survival with transplantation at this point is in the range of 25%. The combined relapse-free survival with chemotherapy alone plus survival with transplantation after first relapse might then be around 50%, i.e. not significantly different from long term disease-free survival for patients transplanted in first remission. However, this is highly speculative since so far no controlled study is available. At the present time it appears that transplantation while in first remission offers the best results. If a patient fails to achieve a first remission or relapses, there is at present little doubt that marrow transplantation offers the best outlook. It should be pointed out, however, that many established transplant centers are reluctant to accept patients in relapse, or assign a relatively low priority (on their waiting lists), which may not be in the patient's best interest.

If no HLA identical donor is available, the situation might be different. However, data reported from a few transplant centers indicate that results with one HLA antigen different transplants might not be different from results obtained with complete HLA identical transplants, especially if the patient is in remission at the time of transplantation. For patients who have a potential donor differing for two HLA antigens or more, transplant should probably not be carried out in first remission, but possibly when the patient suffers a relapse.

Contrary to some of the observations made with congenital disorders, or acquired severe aplastic anemia, transfusion prior to transplantation does not appear to be a major risk factor for the outcome after marrow transplantation.

Acute Lymphoblastic Leukemia (ALL). Although ALL was initially one of the major diagnoses targeted for marrow transplantation, the situation has changed. Several regimens developed in Europe and in the Unites States have achieved complete remissions in more than 90% of patients with ALL. Even a large proportion of high risk patients with B cell, or T lymphoblastic ALL achieve remission. At the present time it appears, therefore, that the low or average risk ALL patient should not be transplanted in first remission, but should be observed for relapse, at least in the pediatric population. Among adults, patients with high risk ALL such as high blast count at diagnosis, mediastinal mass, certain chromosome abnormalities, have a very low probability of long lasting first remission and should be considered for transplant in first remission (see II.2. below).

When treating a patient with ALL, and considering the possibility of subsequent marrow transplantation, one should attempt to avoid CNS toxicity induced by the initial treatment. In particular patients in the pediatric age range who are given cerebro-spinal, or cranial irradiation (usually 1,800 to 2,400 cGy) have an increased risk of developing leukoencephalopathy after transplantation. Toxicity is further increased by the concurrent administration of methotrexate into the spinal canal. Thus, if a patient is a marrow transplant candidate by all other criteria, conceivably one should avoid cranial irradiation and limit CNS treatment and prophylaxis to chemotherapy only. This may be important not only in regards to leukoencephalopathy, but also in regards to growth and development in children. Cranial irradiation, especially if followed later by total body irradiation, clearly impairs growth and psychological development of these patients.

Chronic Myelogenous Leukemia (CML). If a patient is diagnosed as having CML, a donor search should be initiated in all patients, up to about 50 years of age. There is currently no other cure for CML than marrow transplantation. It is more difficult to determine, however, when the transplant should be carried out (see II.2. below).

There are several issues in regards to marrow transplantation for CML which are still unresolved. It appears, however, that prolonged treatment with busulfan may represent a risk factor for marrow transplantation with regards to pulmonary toxicity. Hence, a patient who has been identified as a transplant candidate should preferentially be treated with hydroxyurea rather than busulfan in order to avoid its subsequent impact on marrow transplantation. Another issue is splenomegaly. Although some studies have suggested that splenomegaly is a prognostic indicator, and that splenectomy might improve the outlook in regards to survival and GVHD, this issue is unresolved at the present time (see II.2.). Since these data are evolving constantly, whenever indicated, this issue must be discussed with an expert at a bone marrow transplant center.

Lymphoma. Both Hodgkin's disease and Non-Hodgkin's lymphoma of varying histological subtypes have been treated successfully by marrow transplantation. One might argue that effective curative therapy other than transplantation is available for Hodgkin's disease and for some types of Non-Hodgkin's lymphoma. Nevertheless, some patients should be considered for marrow transplantation, at least when an HLA identical (or one antigen different) donor is available. Patients up to about 40–45 years of age with resistant Hodgkin's disease may benefit from marrow transplantation. In fact, if there is no bone marrow involvement even patients up to 60 years of age could be treated with autologous marrow transplantation.

There are certain sub-categories of Non-Hodgkin's lymphoma with poor prognosis, such as T lymphoblastic or cutaneous lymphoma. These should be considered early on for transplantation if a donor is available. Others have a relatively good prognosis if a first remission can be achieved and would not be immediate transplant candidates (II.2.). Prior irradiation, particularly to the mediastinum, represents a significant risk factor for the postgrafting development of interstitial pneumonitis. Therefore, high dose mediastinal irradiation should be avoided if alternatives are available. Alternatively, the conditioning regimen for marrow transplantation can be modified, such that TBI is not used.

Patient Consultation

As with so many novel treatment approaches, marrow transplantation was initially developed and applied only at a very few centers. No trained physicians were available outside those centers, and patients had little access to information pertaining to this potentially life saving therapy. Since many established and conventionally trained hematologists and oncologists considered the procedure, quite appropriately, experimental, the availability of this modality became known very gradually to only small numbers of patients. Since most of the experience and expertise were limited to a few institutions, patients demanded to be referred there for treatment. Often these patients were not acceptable because, for example, they did not have a suitable donor (see III.1.). Subsequently, however, many referring physicians have taken advantage of the availability of an ever growing expertise in marrow transplantation, and sent patients for a consultation to a transplant center before a decision about marrow transplantation was reached.

This approach has some disadvantages, such as the cost of traveling and a considerable time investment both on the part of the patient and the physician. However, advantages far outweigh disadvantages. Concultation with a physician at a marrow transplant center allows the patient to ask, and more importantly, to obtain answers to questions that could not be well answered elsewhere. It is also possible to provide the patient with recent information not yet published, or publicized. Furthermore, results can be put into perspective better by a transplant physician than by someone not experienced in this field. Very importantly, a patient and any accompanying family member, possibly the potential marrow donor, can visit with patients who are undergoing or recovering from transplantation. This allows insight into the psychological stress and other problems associated with transplantation and often helps the future patient to prepare himself better for transplantation. In addition to the physician's expertise, discussions with nurses and other support personnel are available. Patients can meet a social worker to obtain information regarding other potential problems such as living arrangements, insurance coverage and post-transplant problems. Finally, if the patient indeed is eventually transplanted, and is transplanted at that particular center, he will have familiarized himself already with the environment, and possibly with nurses and physicians who subsequently will be taking care of him. It appears that such an approach reduces the tremendous apprehension and fear associated with marrow transplantation in many patients. This may be due to positive feedback from patients who have gone through the procedure, have done well, and have again developed a positive outlook on life. This often has been crucial for the determination of the patient to proceed with this very involved, expensive treatment, which is still associated with a high probability of morbidity and often mortality.

Where Should a Patient be Transplanted?

In the early and mid 70's there were few bone marrow transplant units operative. Currently there are between 50–100 universities and hospitals in the United States and many others world wide where bone marrow transplantation is being performed. However, this must not be interpreted as an indication that marrow transplantation should be carried out at any hospital where a patient with a disease amenable to transplantation is being diagnosed or treated. Both on financial and scientific grounds, a more limited number of transplant centers is desirable. The resources and support services required for marrow transplantation are considerable, and can be used efficiently and successfully only if a sufficiently large number of patients is undergoing transplantation.

Although from a technical point of view the actual bone marrow transplant is a rather simple procedure, the ramifications of it, and the potential complications associated with it are of considerable complexity. Problems appear to be more severe with more advanced disease, disease duration, patient age and histoincompatible transplants, requiring more expertise and a broader support system. The number of well trained marrow transplant physicians experienced with all aspects of this procedure is limited. As a result many smaller transplant units have carefully selected patients to be transplanted, i.e. have limited transplantation to good risk patients. Poor risk patients, who usually have no other alternative, are referred to larger centers for consideration for transplantation. Obviously, results to be expected in such patients will be poorer than in good risk patients. Thus, one will see reports from small transplant units with results as good or even superior to those reported from larger transplant centers on larger numbers of patients. This can be deceptive. A physician considering referral of a patient for bone marrow transplantation should not be mislead by such statistics.

Even at large transplant centers, however, despite considerable progress many problems remain. Answers to the open questions can be obtained only in controlled studies conducted by experienced investigators and involving sufficiently large numbers of patients. The more efficiently patients are accrued to these studies, the faster answers will be obtained leading to improved survival in future patients. At the same time it is true that many of the larger transplant centers have long waiting lists for patients, and only the better risk patients will be transplanted expeditiously while poorer risk patients will have to wait longer. From a cost/benefit standpoint this is understandable. However, it is of no help to the individual patient. Therefore, a sound approach for any physician taking care of a potential bone marrow transplant candicate would be to call several marrow transplant centers, perhaps one nearby and (if different) one of the large experienced centers, in order to form for himself an opinion as to what the best approach for his patient may be.

References

Appelbaum FR, Clift RA, Buckner CD, Stewart P, Storb R, Sullivan KM, Thomas ED (1983) Allogeneic marrow transplantation for acute nonlymphoblastic leukemia after first relapse. Blood 61: 949

Beatty PG, Clift RA, Mickelson EM, Nisperos BB, Flournoy N, Martin PJ, Sanders JE, Stewart P, Buckner CD, Storb R, Thomas ED, Hansen JA (1985) Marrow transplantation from related donors other than HLA-identical siblings. New Eng J Med 313: 765

Butturini A, Rivera GK, Bortin MM, Gale RP (1987) Which treatment for childhood acute lymphoblastic leukaemia in second remission? The Lancet, I 429

Champlin R, Gale RP (1987) Bone marrow transplantation for acute leukemia: recent advances and comparison with alternative therapies. Seminars in Hematol 24: 55

Doney K, Storb R, Bucker CD, McGuffin R, Witherspoon R, Deeg HJ, Appelbaum FR, Sullivan KM, Thomas EC (1987) Treatment of aplastic anemia with antithymocyte globulin, high-dose corticosteroids, and androgens. Exp Hematol 15: 239

Friedrich W, Goldmann SF, Vetter U, Fliedner TM, Heymer B, Peter HH, Reisner Y, Kleihauer E (1984) Immunoreconstitution in severe combined immunodeficiency after transplantation of HLA-haploidentical, T-cell-depleted bone marrow. The Lancet, I 761

Gluckman E, Berger R, Dutreix J (1984) Bone marrow transplantation for Fanconi anemia. Seminars in Hemat 21: 20

Goldman JM, Apperley JF, Jones L, Marcus R, Goolden WG, Batchelor R, Hale G, Waldmann H, Reid CD, Hows J, Gordon-Smith E, Catovsky D, Galton DAG (1986) Bone marrow transplantation for patients with chronic myeloid leukemia. New Eng J Med 314: 202

Herzig RH, Bortin MM, Barrett AJ, Blume KG, Gluckman E, Horowitz MM, Jacobsen SJ, Marmont A, Masaoka T, Prentice HG, Ramsay NK, Rimm AA, Ringden O, Speck B, Zwaan FE, Gale RP (1987) Bone-marrow transplantation in high-risk acute lymphoblastic leukaemia in first and second remission. The Lancet, I 786

Hoelzer D, Thiel E, Loffler H, Bodenstein H, Plaumann L, Buchner T, Urbanitz D, Koch P, Heimpel H, Engelhardt R, Muller U, Wendt FC, Sodomann H, Ruhl H, Herrmann F, Kaboth W, Dietzfelbinger H, Pralle H, Lunscken Ch, Hellriegel K-P, Spors S, Nowrousian RM, Fischer J, Fulle H, Mitrou PS, Pfreundschuh M, Gorg Ch, Emmerich B, Queisser W, Meyer P, Labedzki L, Essers U, Konig H, Mainzer K, Herrmann R, Messerer D, Zwingers T (1984) Intensified therapy in acute lymphoblastic and acute undifferentiated leukemia in adults. Blood 64: 38

Lucarelli G, Izzi T, Porcellini A, Delfini C, Galimberti M, Polchi P, Moretti L, Manna A, Sparaventi G (1983) Fetal liver transplant in aplastic anemia and acute leukemia. Recent Advances in Bone Marrow Transplantation R.P. Gale (ed.) Alan R. Liss, Inc. New York pp. 865

O'Leary M, Ramsay NK, Nesbit ME, Hurd D, Woods WG, Krivit W, Kim TH, McGlave P, Kersey J (1983) Bone marrow transplantation for non-Hodgkin's lymphoma in children and yound adults. Am J of Med 74: 497

Phillips GL, Herzig RH, Lazarus HM, Fay JW, Wolff SN, Mill WB, Lin HS, Thomas PR, Glasgow GP, Shina DC, Herzig GP (1984) Treatment of resistant malignant lymphoma with cyclophosphamide, total body irradiation, and transplantation of cryopreserved autologous marrow. New Eng J Med 310: 1157

Preisler H, Davis RB, Kirshner J, Dupre E, Richards F, Hoagland HC, Kopel S, Levy RN, Carey R, Schulman P, Gottlieb AJ, McIntyre OR, and the Cancer and Leukemia Group B (1987) Comparison of three remission induction regimens and two postinduction strategies for the treatment of acute nonlymphocytic leukemia: a cancer and leukemia group B study. Blood, 69: 1441

Rivera GK, Buchanan G, Boyett JM, Camitta B, Ochs J, Kalwinsky D, Amylon M, Vietti TJ, Crist WM (1986) Intensive retreatment of childhood acute lymphoblastic leukemia in first bone marrow relapse. New Eng J Med 315: 273

Santos GW, Tutschka PJ, Brookmeyer R, Saral R, Beschorner WE, Bias WB, Braine HG, Burns WH, Elfenbein GJ, Kaizer H, Mellits D, Sensenbrenner LL, Stuart RK, Yeager AM (1983) Marrow transplantation for acute nonlymphocytic leukemia after treatment with busulfan and cyclophosphamide. New Eng J Med 309: 1347

Speck B, Gratwohl A, Nissen C, Osterwalder B, Wursch A, Tichelli A, Lori A, Reusser P, Jeannet M, Signer E (1986) Treatment of severe aplastic anemia. Exp Hematol 14: 126

Storb R, Thomas ED, Buckner CD, Appelbaum FR, Clift RA, Deeg HJ, Doney K, Hansen JA, Prentice RL, Sanders JE, Stewart P, Sullivan KM, Witherspoon RP (1984) Marrow transplan tation for aplastic anemia. Seminars in Hemat 21: 27

Thomas ED (1983) Marrow transplantation for malignant diseases. (Karnofsky Memorial Lecture) J Clin Oncol 1: 517

Thomas ED, Clift RA, Fefer A, Appelbaum FR, Beatty P, Bensinger WI, Buckner D, Cheever MA, Deeg HJ, Doney K, Flournoy N, Greenberg P, Hansen JA, Martin P, McGuffin R, Ramberg R, Sanders JE, Singer J, Stewart P, Storb R, Sullivan K, Weiden PL, Witherspoon R (1986) Marrow transplantation for the treatment of chronic myelogenous leukemia. Ann Int Med 104: 155

Touraine JL (1983) European experience with fetal tissue transplantation in severe combined immunodeficiency. Birth Defects 19: 139

Weinstein HJ, Mayer RJ, Rosenthal DS, Coral FS, Camitta BM, Gelber RD (1983) Chemotherapy for acute myelogenous leukemia in children and adults: VAPA update. Blood 62: 315

2. When Should Marrow Transplantation be Considered?

Marrow transplantation, once a salvage procedure for patients with resistant and end-stage leukemia is now generally performed much earlier in the patient's disease course. While in remission, almost all patients are in good physical condition, well able to tolerate the impact of the preparative regimen. Furthermore, tumor cells may not be as resistant to chemotherapy as in later stages. Improved survival for patients transplanted in remission is due to fewer deaths from non-leukemic causes, and to fewer deaths from relapse following transplant.

The patient's *age* plays a major role in the decision making process of marrow transplantation. Several studies have shown that the risk of developing post-transplant complications increases with age. This is particularly true for acute GVHD. The problem of more severe acute GVHD becomes most prominent in patients over 45–50 years of age, and the incidence of septic complications and of idiopathic interstitial pneumonitis increases substantially in this age group. Consequently, most transplant centers have set the age limit for allogeneic marrow grafting at 45–50 years. However, an occasional patient in good clinical condition might be considered for a transplant even over 50 years of age. Older patients least likely to suffer transplant related complications are those patients with minimal pre-treatment history, and those with minimal or no problems other than their underlying illness. Pulmonary and cardiac function studies may be used to assess these conditions when appropriate. Non-smokers and patients in good physical condition appear to tolerate the transplant procedure better. Recent data indicate that allogeneic marrow transplantation for diseases such as CML in chronic phase and preleukemia may have a better prognosis relative to age than marrow grafting for patients with acute myelogenous or lymphoblastic leukemia in the same age range. Therefore, the decision to transplant or not must be made on an individual basis. The following discussion is meant to provide guidelines for timing of allogeneic marrow transplantation in different diseases. Indications for autologous transplantation are discussed where appropriate.

Severe Aplastic Anemia

Marrow transplantation is the treatment of choice for patients with aplastic anemia, provided an HLA identical donor is available. Transplantation should be performed as soon as possible after diagnosis to prevent sensitization of the recipient by multiple transfusions that might otherwise be required. This is important as graft rejection occurs more frequently in those patients who receive transfusions before marrow transplantation. The number of transfusions in particular is a risk factor for marrow graft rejection. Platelets are generally contaminated with leukocytes which express both class I (HLA A and B) and class II (HLA D, DR) antigens on their surface, and have been shown to provide a very potent stimulus in sensitizing the recipient. In an untransfused patient, the probability of becoming a long term survivor is about 80–90% while transfused patients have a probability of survival of about 60–70%.

Nevertheless, since it is time consuming to identify a potential donor, to perform HLA-typing and mixed lymphocyte cultures, and to find a transplant center which will be able to accept the patient, it is likely that the patient will require transfusions. During this time, platelet transfusions should be given only therapeutically in case of hemorrhagic complications and not on a prophylactic basis. Conceivably, platelets from single donors may be preferable to prevent sensitization of the patient against a broad spectrum of HLA antigens. However, family members must *not* be used for platelet donation before marrow transplantation in order to avoid exposure of the patient to histocompatibility antigens that might also be expressed on marrow cells from the marrow donor. If red blood cell transfusions are necessary, leukocyte-poor (buffy-coat depleted) preparations should be given. In addition, longer storage times for red blood cells can decrease the stimulatory ability of leukocytes. Thus, a cautious transfusion policy in patients with aplastic anemia can help reduce sensitization of the recipient and reduce the risk of graft rejection and associated transplant related mortality.

Treatment of severe aplastic anemia with antihymocyte globulin (ATG) represents an alternative approach in patients for whom no HLA-genotypically or phenotypically matched related marrow donor is available. In some studies response rates to ATG therapy range from 40–60%, although frequently hematopoetic reconstitution is not complete, and laboratory investigations indicate that hematopoesis remains abnormal in nearly all patients so treated. ATG treatment should be considered as first line therapy for all patients for whom only an HLA-mismatched donor is available. However, if a repeated course of ATG has been unsuccessful, marrow transplantation may be considered even in the mismatched situation, particularly in young patients. This has to be considered a salvage procedure since the risk of graft rejection and severe acute graft-versus-host disease is substantial. Under these circumstances, again, a prudent transfusion policy will improve the prognosis with marrow transplantation if performed at some later time.

Acute Myelocytic Leukemia

Patients with acute myelocytic leukemia (AML), who have an HLA-identical donor, have the best prognosis when transplanted in first remission. Data indicate that the probability of long term survival is 40–60% for those transplanted in first remission. If marrow grafting cannot be done in first remission, transplantation in first relapse may be preferable to second remission. The corresponding data for first relapse and second remission in a retrospective analysis were about 35% and 25% respectively. Apparently, the additional chemotherapy needed to achieve another remission is harmful to the patient and increases transplant related complications such as veno-occlusive disease and interstitial pneumonitis. Relapse rate, however, is the same in both groups.

Recent studies have shown that results with transplants from family donors who differ for only one HLA antigen are not different from those in patients with HLA-genotypically or phenotypically identical donors. Therefore, the timing of marrow transplantation for this group of patients should be the same as for those having an HLA-identical donor. The results obtained with more severely mismatched related donors (2 or 3 HLA-antigens different) are inferior, and presumably not better than those obtained with chemotherapy alone. Consequently, the approach has generally been not to transplant these patients at all, or only if and when their disease progresses, i.e. after the first relapse, at a time when chemotherapy no longer offers a realistic alternative. Furthermore, encouraging results have been achieved with autologous transplantation in first or even second remission. To date, no statistically significant difference in disease-free survival has been demonstrated for autologous marrow purged of tumor cells as compared to unpurged marrow. On the other hand, allogeneic transplantation in the two or three antigen mismatchend situation or from an unrelated donor might be considered as salvage treatment in second or later remission. Some centers, however, prefer to transplant a patient with marrow from an unrelated donor even in first remission if no genotypically identical (related) donor is available.

Children with AML should also be transplanted in first remission if an HLA-identical donor is available. The probability of long-term survival for these patients is 60–70%, i.e. superior to the best reported results with intensive maintenance chemotherapy. Due to insufficient data, it is not clear at present when a one antigen mismatched related, a matched unrelated, or an autologous transplant should be performed in these patients.

Preleukemia

Patients with preleukemia, particularly those with de novo preleukemia and without severe marrow fibrosis, should be transplanted shortly after diagnosis if an HLA-identical donor is available. Relapse rate in these patients is extremely low, when an appropriate conditioning regimen including total body irradiation is employed. Since marrow morphology cannot always clearly distinguish between preleukemia and aplastic anemia, cytogenetic analysis should be performed in each patient. Patients who have extensive marrow fibrosis do poorly secondary to graft failure. Patients who develop secondary preleukemia after previous anticancer treatment also have a less favorable prognosis. These facts should be considered when making a decision as to when to transplant a patient with preleukemia.

Acute Lymphoblastic Leukemia

Adult patients with newly diagnosed ALL can be subdivided into high and low risk groups. Assignment to the high risk group is based on the following criteria:
- White blood cell count $>30 \times 10^9$/L at diagnosis
- Phenotype of blast cells: B or null
- Slow to achieve first complete remission
- Age of patient
- Presence of a mediastinal mass at diagnosis
- CNS involvement at presentation

It is recommended that patients who belong to this "high risk" group receive an allogeneic transplant in first remission, provided an HLA-identical, or a one antigen mismatched related donor is available. Patients who do not have an appropriate donor may qualify for an unrelated or autologous transplant performed in first remission. Patients with a two or even three antigen mismatched donor may be considered for an allogeneic transplant in second or subsequent remission, especially when they are young (<20 years). In older patients, mismatched transplants are associated with a high mortality rate and represent a last treatment option.

For "low risk" patients, current therapeutic protocols with chemotherapy only offer long term disease free survival of 40–60%. However, when these patients relapse, second and subsequent remissions are usually short-lived with a median duration of about 6 months. No curative conventional approach can be offered to these patients and, therefore, marrow transplantation should be considered in second or subsequent remission even from a mismatched related or a phenotypically matched unrelated donor.

Although the data on autologous marrow transplantation in patients with ALL are not yet conclusive, this modality can be entertained as an alternative approach especially if the patient is older (>20 years) and only mismatched donors are available for allogeneic marrow grafting.

The situation in *children* is slightly different in so far as current treatment protocols promise long term survival even in children with less favourable prognosis. However, allogeneic transplantation is strongly recommended for those patients who relapse while receiving appropriate maintainance chemotherapy or in children with testicular or CNS relapse once another remission is achieved. Furthermore, L3 morphology (Burkitt type) or the presence of a Philadelphia chromosome are associated with poor prognosis with conventional chemotherapy and such patients should be considered candidates for marrow grafting in first remission.

No firm recommendation can be given for children with low risk disease. It appears reasonable to transplant these patients, as adults, in second remission. This view might be challenged, however, by some investigators who have achieved excellent chemotherapy results with disease-free survival in excess of 50% in children who were induced into a second remission.

Chronic Myelogenous Leukemia

Patients with CML who have an HLA-identical donor should be transplanted while in chronic phase. Recent studies have shown that results are best if marrow transplantation is performed early after diagnosis. It is not clear yet if the inferior prognosis in patients transplanted later is directly related to prolonged treatment with busulfan which may render the lungs, and possibly other organs, more susceptible to transplant related complications. However, because of these presumed negative effects, it appears advisable to omit busulfan in patients in chronic phase and instead use hydroxyurea to control leukocytosis.

It has also been shown that post transplant prognosis for those patients who, following blast transformation, can achieve a second chronic phase with conventional chemotherapy is superior to the outlook with transplantation in blast transformation. This advantage seems more often to be associated with the lymphoblastic type of CML blast crisis. Thus, it may be useful to phenotype blast cells early if they are lymphoblastic, and attempt to achieve a second chronic phase with standard chemotherapy before proceeding to marrow grafting.

Autologous transplantation in CML has been studied primarily in patients who have entered blast crisis. These patients were treated with high dose chemoradiotherapy, and had their marrow harvested while in "remission" and stored for subsequent transplant. However, remission duration was short in almost all patients, and most centers have abandoned this technique. Another treatment option for patients who do not have an HLA-identical donor may soon become available: autologous marrow reinfusion after in vitro long term culture of the bone marrow (see III.3.). Under certain circumstances, malignant cells die earlier in cell cultures than normal cells, which can then be harvested and reinfused into the patient. If this technique proves to be effective, it may open new perspectives in autografting for patients with CML.

A number of patients in chronic phase will have an enlarged spleen. The question arises as to whether splenectomy should be performed in these patients before transplantation or not. The data so far fail to show any significant effect of splenectomy on survival or on recurrence of leukemia. However, platelet transfusion support is easier after splenectomy. Therefore, this procedure is recommended for patients with large spleens in whom mechanical problems are encountered or in whom difficulties in platelet transfusion support after transplantation are anticipated.

Malignant Lymphoma

Despite substantial progress in the treatment of malignant lymphomas with conventional modalities, some patients relapse and eventually become resistant to conventional chemo-radiotherapy. Marrow transplantation in these refractory cases has met with only limited success, and consequently attemps have been made to identify high risk patients that may benefit from marrow grafting.

Involvement of the CNS, the bone marrow or both at the time of diagnosis in patients with non-Hodgkin's lymphoma has been shown to be associated with early relapse and poor survival. Lymphoblastic lymphomas of the convoluted cell type also have a very poor prognosis with conventional chemotherapy alone. Therefore, in these patients, allogeneic marrow transplantation should be considered in first remission, if the patient has an HLA-identical donor. Moreover, patients who do not achieve a complete remission or relapse early after a full course of first line chemotherapy are also candidates for marrow grafting. Some studies indicate that patients with advanced Hodgkin's disease who relapse within the first year after initiating treatment should be considered for transplantation, since their survival with conventional chemotherapy is poor.

Autologous transplantation in malignant lymphoma is receiving increasing attention, especially in cases where no obvious marrow involvement can be demonstrated. However, no sensitive tests are available yet to exclude this possibility with complete certainty.

About 70% of all patients with high grade non-Hodgkin's lymphoma who achieve a complete remission with conventional chemotherapy survive 5 years or longer. Thus, autologous transplantation is not justified as consolidation treatment in general and should be reserved for patients in the high risk group defined above. Those patients who fail after a full course of first line chemotherapy are also candidates for autologous marrow grafting, if their marrow is histologically normal. Longterm disease-free survival for such patients, however, is probably no better than 30% at present.

Prior chest (mediastinal) irradiation in patients with malignant lymphoma is associated with an increased incidence of fatal interstitial pneumonia after marrow grafting. Therefore, in a newly diagnosed patient with malignant lymphoma, omitting chest irradiation from the initial treatment approach should be considered if it will not affect immediate prognosis. Alternatively, a conditioning regimen without total body irradiation (e.g. high dose etoposide and thiotepa) may be selected for marrow grafting.

Multiple Myeloma

Although most patients with this disease are more than 50 years of age, an occasional younger patient is affected by multiple myeloma which can progress rapidly despite chemotherapy. The clinical experience with marrow transplantation in multiple myeloma is still very limited. However, transplantation should be considered in patients under 50 years of age if an HLA-identical marrow donor is available and the disease progresses on conventional treatment such as melphalan and prednisone.

Alternatively, for those patients without a suitable donor, and particularly for older patients, autologous stem cell transplantation (see III.3.) is currently being evaluated. Since multiple myeloma usually does not present with malignant cells in the peripheral blood, this treatment option appears to be a promising approach. Autologous marrow transplantation is not considered appropriate as histologically normal remission marrow is unusual in myeloma with current regimens and successful purging techniques for autologous marrow in this disease are not yet available.

Congenital disorders

A variety of otherwise fatal genetic disease have been treated successfully by marrow transplantation (Table 2). Since almost all these disorders are lethal in the first or second decade of life, transplantation should be performed as early as possible to prevent debilitating sequelae of the disease and to minimize the risk intrinsic to the procedure. Long-term disease-free survival exceeds 90% in those patients who are transplanted before the onset of major infections. Furthermore, transfusion products sensitize the patient and may hamper successful engraftment later.

One of the most common genetic disorders worldwide is β-thalassemia. The homozygous form is a serious disease which can become life-threatening mainly because of the numerous blood transfusions necessary to maintain an adequate hemoglobin level. Iron overload and subsequent organ failure are common. Allogeneic marrow transplantation can cure a significant proportion of these patients. Pooled date from several centers show survival of about 75% with about 55% of all grafted patients free of thalassemia.

When deciding to transplant these patients one has to consider that some patients would have lived for some time with conventional treatment. The question as to when an allogeneic transplant in a patient with homozygous thalassemia is indicated clearly has to be answered on an individual basis: those who can be provided life long transfusion and chelation therapy, and who are also willing to cope with this cumbersome treatment, should be managed by conventional treatment. However, patients with an HLA-identical marrow donor should be offered a transplant if these conditions are not met. Marrow transplantation is then best carried out early in life, since transfusion-induced sensitization influences survival rate.

Solid Tumors

The treatment of selected solid tumors with autologous transplantation is still largely experimental, and no cures have been reported. However, this may change with more effective and selective chemotherapeutic agents. Autologous transplantation is currently being studied in patients with testicular carcinoma, breast cancer, glioblastoma, lung cancer, neuroblastoma und melanoma.

References

Appelbaum FR (1987) Hammering away at solid tumors. Canc Treat Rep, 71: 115

Appelbaum FR, Storb R, Ramberg RE et al (1987) Treatment of preleukemia syndromes with marrow transplantation. Blood 69: 92

Blume KG, Forman SJ, Snyder DS et al (1987) Allogeneic bone marrow transplantation for acute lymphoblastic leukemia during first complete remission. Transplantation 43: 389

Deeg HJ, Self S, Storb R, Doney K, Appelbaum, FR, Witherspoon RP, Sullivan KM, Sheehan K, Sanders J, Mickelson E, Thomas ED (1986) Decreased incidence of marrow graft rejection in patients with severe aplastic anemia: changing impact of risk factors. Blood 68: 1363

Klingemann HG, Self S, Banaji M et al (1987) Refractoriness to random donor platelet transfusions in patients with aplastic anaemia: a multivariate analysis of data from 264 cases. Br J Haematol 66: 115

Klingemann HG, Storb R, Fefer A et al (1986) Bone marrow transplantation in patients aged 45 years and older. Blood 67: 770

O'Reilly RJ, Brochstein J, Dinsmore R, Kirkpatric D (1984) Marrow transplantation for congenital disorders. Sem Hematol 1041: 155

Sullivan KM, Appelbaum FR, Horning ST et al Selection of patients with Hodgkin's disease and non-Hodgkin's lymphoma for bone marrow transplantation. Int J Cell Clon 4: 94 (Suppl. 1)

Thomas ED, Clift RA, Fefer A et al (1986) Marrow transplantation for the treatment of chronic myelogenous leukemia. Ann Int Med 21: 188

Tura S (1986) Bone marrow transplantation in multiple myeloma: currrent status and future perspectives. Bone Marrow Transplantation 1: 17

3. Preparation for Marrow Transplantation

This section deals with the mechanics of preparing for marrow transplantation. Some patients will be evaluated by the Transplant Team before the results of tests that indicate eligibility for transplantation are available, while other patients will arrive at the Transplant Center with all test results known, and having been fully informed of the procedure. In any case, it is necessary to discuss with the patient the important aspects of transplantation shortly before the conditioning regimen begins. An overall schema of this procedure is offered in Table 4. (Since most transplants are from normal donors, this approach is emphasized. However, the use and indeed desirability of autologous marrow transplantation is discussed below.)

Discussion with the Patient

The initial visit should be simple and straightforward, as it is important to remember that when patients are first evaluated by the Transplant Team, they may have widely-varying amounts of information regarding marrow transplantation. The ability of many patients to absorb large quantities of unfamiliar data during an initial (and often stressful) visit is limited. Therefore, subsequent discussions, pamphlets and audio-visual materials are helpful. Patients and families often appreciate being given a tour of the Transplant Unit and the opportunity to meet other members of staff (especially nursing personnel) during their initial visit.

The initial discussion session may begin with a review of the patient's diagnosis, disease status and natural history. Next, the reasons for considering marrow transplantation are detailed, specifically the rationale of marrow transplantation in general and for the particular disease considered.

The prognosis after marrow transplantation must be compared in detail with that for other treatment options. This is particularly important for patients for whom marrow transplantation is not the only potentially curative option, e.g., those with acute leukemia in the initial remission. Although it is very unlikely that a member of the Transplant Team would deliberately mislead a patient, the mere fact of his or her enthusiasm for marrow transplantation might subtly influence a patient to accept marrow transplantation rather than more conventional therapy. This situation is particularly undesirable because marrow trans-

Table 4. Patient Preparation for Marrow Transplantation

A)	Discussion of marrow transplantation, including its rationale, risks, and benefits to the patient, family and referring physician. (Particular attention must be devoted to discussing alternative therapies.)
B)	Complete medical history, including: 1. Unequivocal confirmation of diagnosis 2. Previous treatment 3. Specific disease or treatment-related problems 4. Transfusions 5. Co-morbid medical problems 6. Allergies 7. Psychologic assessment
C)	Histocompatibility testing for allogeneic and syngeneic marrow transplantation 1. Serologic typing on patient and nuclear (or extended) family 2. Mixed leukocyte testing on the patient and prospective donor
D)	Transfusion support planning in all patients: 1. Evaluation of allosensitization status 2. ABO typing of patient and donor
E)	Determination of marker of engraftment for allogeneic marrow transplantation
F)	Toxicity screening: 1. Pertinent history 2. Serum tests of renal, hepatic, and endocrine function 3. Pulmonary function tests including arterial blood gases and diffusing capacity of carbon monoxide (DLCO) 4. Left ventricular function evaluation 5. Creatinine clearance
G)	Tumor staging studies for malignant diseases 1. Bone marrow biopsy 2. Central nervous system 3. Sanctuary sites 4. Others as required
H)	Sperm banking

plantation is currently plagued by high intrinsic morbidity and mortality rates. Finally, although the chief reason for considering a marrow transplant is cure, some patients arrive with the misconception that marrow transplantation is invariably curative. This idea must be dispelled.

It is most important that the immediate and delayed toxicities of marrow transplantation are detailed, including the acute side effects of the conditioning regimen and the period of debility and hospitalization before engraftment. The important complications of graft-vs-host disease (GVHD) and interstitial pneumonitis must be discussed fully. Although fatal toxicities are more obvious, it is important to discuss the possibility of persistent debilities of a non-fatal nature, such as chronic GVHD. Other late complications should also be discussed, especially the possibility of second malignancy (currently a problem more theoretical than actual). Also, it is important to raise the issue of sterility; this complication is likely in patients receiving more intensive conditioning, and often is not considered by patients.

Discussion with the Potential Donor

It is likely that some potential donors do not exercise any real choice in the donation of marrow for transplantation, as it is usually assumed that they will participate. Of course, this should not be assumed; an informed potential donor who truly does not wish to donate marrow should be supported in this decision. More commonly, potential donors are eager to participate but often have concerns that they may be reluctant to voice, e.g., they may fear anesthesia or needles, or have a history of certain social habits with major medical consequences, e.g. homosexuality or intravenous drug use. We find that potential donors must be asked specifically about these matters, as well as about their concerns regarding the procedure itself, preferably not with the donor and other family members present.

It is also helpful to make at least a superficial psychological assessment of the potential donor. While it is unlikely that a potential donor would have an occult psychiatric disorder of such magnitude as to lead to something as catastrophic as the withdrawal of their participation at a critical time, this is certainly possible. In addition, a donor may take on an inappropriate burden of guilt for an unsuccessful transplant. When psychologic dysfunction is suspected, consultation is recommended.

Role of the Referring Physician

After the referring physician has given preliminary consideration to the patient's suitability for marrow transplantation, consulting with the Transplant Team by telephone is often the most convenient method of initiating contact (see II, 1). During this contact, the potential risks and benefits of marrow transplantation should be discussed, and a preliminary decision regarding the patient's suitability should be reached.

The referring physician plays a key role in preparing a potential patient and donor for marrow transplantation. In addition to helping to assess the medical suitability of the procedure, the referring physician may be able to point out important non-medical considerations, (e.g., unusual family interactions) that could have bearing on the case.

If the referring physician and the Transplant Team decide to proceed with a formal evaluation, it is most helpful if the physician transmits to the Team the patient's complete medical history as well as initial histocompatibility data. However, certain Transplant Centers prefer to perform some or all of the histocompatibility studies themselves, and it is important to be aware of this to avoid expensive duplication. Depending on bed availability, the referral process may be expedited if the physician additionally performs tumor staging studies, baseline organ toxicity determinations and a medical evaluation of the donor. Again, the Transplant Center should be consulted in this regard.

Role of the Transplant Team

It is vital that from the onset frank communication be established between the Transplant Team and the patient, family and referring physician. This is especially important because marrow transplantation is radical therapy, and few patients are fully aware of the potential adverse consequences. Also, the Transplant Team member consulted should be capable of accurately discussing in detail other (i.e., non-transplant) treatment options. If this is not the case, an appropriate consultation to discuss such options should be obtained promptly.

Patients must often wait some time before a bed is available in the Transplant Unit. It is desirable for the Transplant Team to assume primary management in this interval, as such an arrangement initiates the relationship with the Team member and ensures that any interim therapeutic measures will not conflict with the transplantation schedule.

Medical Evaluation

It is obvious that a complete history and physical exam is required on the patient. The following points deserve special emphasis.

Confirmation of Diagnosis

While this point is so apparent that its inclusion may seem superfluous, some patients arrive at the Transplant Center with no evidence of disease (i.e., those in remission). Although it is unlikely that the referring physician has made a major error in diagnosis, all tissues obtained in previous diagnostic studies should be reviewed by a pathologist who works closely with the Transplant Team. If any questions arise, additional specimens from previous tissue sections, or repeat biopsy procedures may be required. Also, even a lesser discrepancy (e.g., a misclassification of the type of acute leukemia) may be important, as many Transplant Centers have different conditioning regimens for the various types of leukemia.

Previous Treatment

This point is important for two reasons. First, the level of response to prior therapy, e.g. the history of a previous remission with conventional antileukemic chemotherapy, may provide vital information about prognosis after transplantation or dictate changes in the transplant regimen. Second, cumulative toxicity potentially produced by such therapy might pose excessive hazards after transplantation. The Transplant Team needs to be aware, for example, of the cumulative doses of anthracyclines, cis-platin, bleomycin and radiation, as well as any evidence of toxicity of these agents (see below).

Disease-related Problems

For Patients who have active disease, it is important to know the sites and extent of disease, for its bearing not only on prognosis but also regarding the use of adjunctive special therapies (e.g., local radiotherapy to nodes obstructing vital structures or to testicular tumors and intrathecal chemotherapy).

Co-morbid Medical Problems

A close history and subsequent evaluation concerning this aspect should be performed. Specifically, a previous history of cardiac, renal, endocrine or hepatic disease must be solicited, as damage to any one of the organs involved may complicate transplantation (see below).

Transfusions

Specifics concerning the number, type, result and reactions to previous transfusions with all blood components must be obtained. This information could influence the type of conditioning, or indicate the desirability of one (histocompatible) donor over another. Likewise, a history of pregnancy in female patients must be elicited.

Allergies

Although a history of documented or probable allergies are part of the routine history, special attention should be directed to those agents which the patient will almost inevitably receive posttransplant, e.g., penicillins, trimethoprim-sulfamethoxazole, and allopurinol.

Psychologic Assessment

Some centers prefer routine psychologic screening of all patients. This may be desirable, but is probably unnecessary. However, a previous history of psychologic instability or a psychiatric diagnosis must be fully delineated. Continuation of established liaisons between the patient and a psychiatrist or psychologist may be helpful during the posttransplant period. Moreover, an unrealistic or otherwise inappropriate attitude towards the transplant procedure probably should also be evaluated formally.

Most patients considering a therapy as drastic as marrow transplantation have an appropriate degree of anxiety. However, it is necessary to distinguish these patients from others who enter the marrow transplantation procedure with less than a full commitment. Patients in the latter group may be expected to respond poorly to information concerning unexpected complications and related requests for invasive procedures (e.g., open lung biopsy for interstitial pneumonitis). Identifying these patients and obtaining psychiatric consultation for them is vital.

Histocompatibility Evaluation for Routine Allogeneic Marrow Transplantation

When a patient is referred to a Transplant Center, histocompatibility testing of the human leukocyte antigen (HLA) complex for the HLA-A and -B alleles of the patient and (at least some) family members will generally have been performed. It is also necessary to test for the alleles at the HLA-D/DR locus in the patient and prospective donor(s). If this typing has not been performed, or if, in the assessment of the Transplant Team, there is any question about its accuracy, tissue typing should be repeated at the Transplant Center. Furthermore, it may be necessary to perform such typing in additional family members (e.g., parents, children) to delineate genotypic as opposed to phenotypic matching (Fig. 1A and B).

A number of variables potentially complicate satisfactory HLA typing. For instance, HLA-D/DR typing may be inaccurate in certain circumstances, i.e., with relapsed acute leukemia, chronic myelogenous leukemia (CML), and aplastic anemia, as well as in patients who have recently received chemotherapy or transfusions. Therefore, in patients with malignancy, tissue typing should ideally be performed when the primary disease is under satisfactory control and several weeks after chemotherapy has ended. For patients receiving intermittent courses of chemotherapy this is usually not difficult, while for those requiring continuous chemotherapy or with nonremitting diseases (e.g., aplastic anemia or CML) this may pose a problem. In patients with CML in particular, it is often very difficult to obtain satisfactory D/DR typing. In this situation it may be possible to use chemotherapy (usually hydroxyurea) to lower the leukocyte count to $<10.0 \times 10^9/L$, to discontinue therapy for several days to weeks, then to repeat the D/DR typing before the leukocyte count rebounds. However, this method is not foolproof and adequate D/DR typing simply may not be possible in some cases of CML.

Satisfactory tissue typing is obviously essential. A member of the Transplant Team should be consulted concerning the timing or other specifics of the HLA testing whenever any question exists.

Suitable Normal Donors for Marrow Transplantation

Syngeneic Donors

Except for the lack of a possible graft-vs-leukemia effect, an identical twin is an ideal donor for several reasons:

a) In some cases, the contitioning regimen may be selected to avoid immunosuppression, and occasionally conditioning is not even required (some cases of aplastic anemia);

b) Rejection and graft-vs-host disease do not occur, and cytomegalovirus (CMV) interstitial pneumonitis is infrequent; and
c) The toxicities of therapies for these problems are avoided. However, one must insure that a patient and donor are indeed genetically identical as much as possible, as altered conditioning regimens and the deletion of graft-vs-host disease prophylaxis may be disastrous in non-identical twins.

The following studies are suggested to this end: general physical phenotype, dermatographics, HLA typing, and complete erythrocyte phenotype typing. An obstetric record of a monozygotic placenta is desirable.

Allogeneic Donors

Providing standard disease and disease status indications are present, allogeneic marrow transplantation can be routinely recommended when histocompatible related donors, either genotypically HLA-identical siblings (Fig. 1A) or phenotypically identical family members (Fig. 1B), are available. Approximately

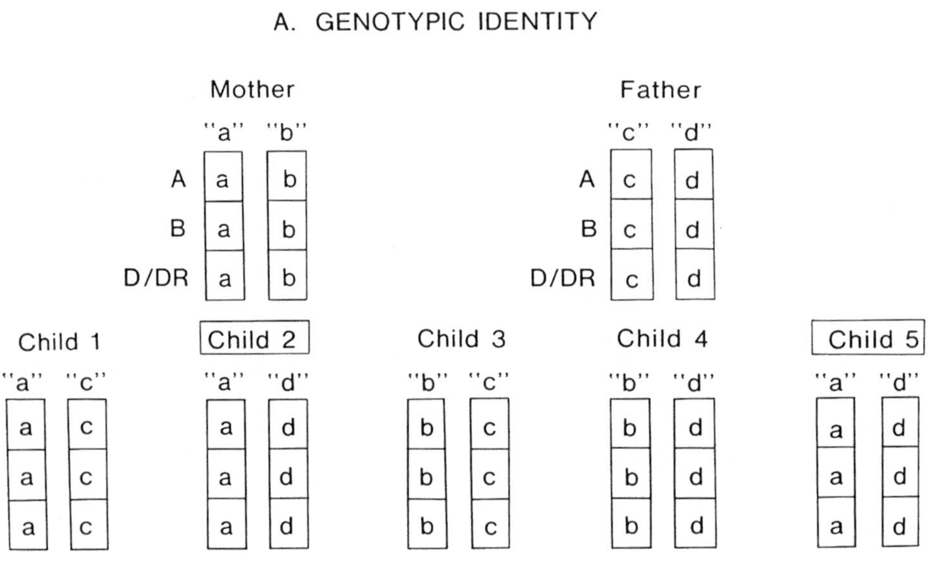

Fig. 1A–C. Inheritance of HLA Antigens in a family. **A)** Paternal and maternal chromosomes were inherited by the children such that children 2 and 5 are genotypically identical for HLA; **B)** The father is homozygous for the HLA antigens, and either one of the two paternal chromosomes will confer the same phenotype to the children. Consequently, children 3 and 5 (and children 2 and 4) are phenotypically HLA identical. Only if additional markers (located on chromosome 6) differ between the two paternal chromosomes can genotypic identity be determined (such a determination may also be possible using restriction fragment length polymorphism for certain DNA sequences within HLA); **C)** Children 2 and 5 have inherited the same maternal chromosome (a) but differ for D/DR antigens on the paternal chromosome. Such a situation can be due to a cross-over event during meiosis such that a segment of one chromosome is exchanged with the corresponding segment from the second chromosome. In this example the result is a one antigen mismatch involving the D/DR region

25–40% of patients will have the former source of donor marrow, while the latter is quite uncommon. The use of patient and donor pairs with minimal histoincompatibility (i.e., sharing of one haplotype [chromosome] plus incompatibility only at a single allele on the non-shared chromosome, either HLA-A, -B, -D or -DR (Fig. 1C) may be considered with good-risk patients, such as leukemic patients in remission or stable phase. Such donors are relatively uncommon, and are identified for only 5–10% of prospective patients. In all other situations involving a more severe degree of mismatch at HLA, allogeneic marrow transplantation must be considered experimental.

B. AN EXAMPLE OF PHENOTYPIC IDENTITY

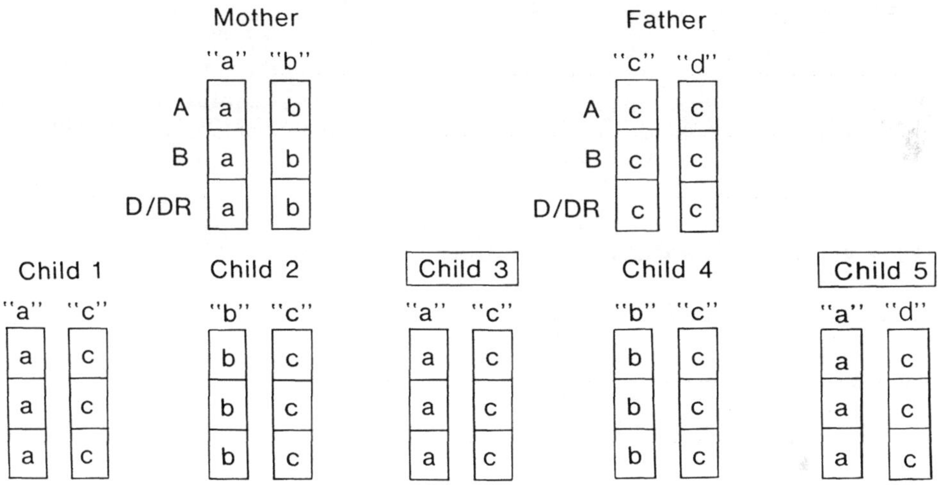

C. ONE- ANTIGEN MISMATCH

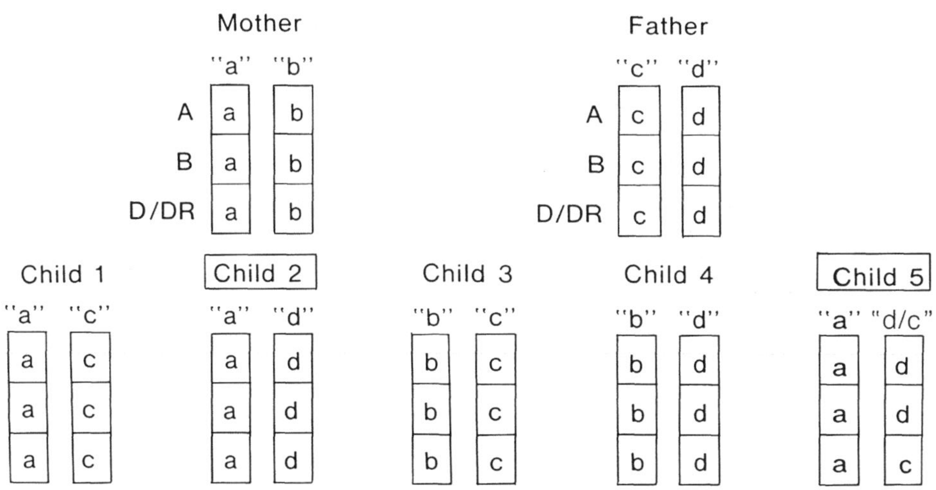

Occasionally, when an HLA-identical sibling is not available, the question of typing members of the extended family arises. In general, this is not a fruitful endeavor, but it may be considered in some situations in which a transplant is highly desirable (e.g., a young patient with CML), when there is an abundance of extended family members available, and the resources for the expense of such typing exist.

For allogeneic marrow transplantation, identifying a marker of engraftment is highly desirable. Sex chromosome or erythrocyte phenotypic differences are currently the most commonly used methods. In future, the use of molecular genetic techniques such as restriction fragment length polymorphisms (RFLP) will likely become standard.

Donor Preference

Due to their lack of complications, syngeneic transplants are virtually always preferred, but of course this is a very rare option. Although in most instances an HLA-identical related donor is unavailable, the opposite situation will occasionally arise, i.e., more than one histocompatible donor will be identified.

Other Potential Sources of Donor Marrow

Autologous Marrow Transplantation

Overview

The current requirement for a reasonably normal marrow status at the time of harvest largely limits autologous marrow transplantation to being a "rescue" procedure for certain cancer patients undergoing intensive cytotoxic therapy. A related potential use is the cryopreservation of autologous marrow for high-risk nuclear workers. This suggestion is offered in light of the Chernobyl nuclear disaster, in which some patients required marrow transplants. Unfortunately, it was difficult to obtain adequate HLA-typing of these pancytopenic patients, thus greatly hindering the identification of suitable allogeneic donors. (Even without this problem, the number of patients with suitable donors would be low.) Although the cost of autologous marrow harvest, cryopreservation and long-term storage would be substantial, the proven ability of cryopreserved autologous marrow to reconstitute hematopoiesis after marrow-lethal therapy without rejection or graft-vs-host disease makes it an attractive alternative to allogeneic marrow in this situation. Finally, if gene therapy procedures become practical, autologous marrow transplantation may potentially be applicable to certain congenital immunohematologic disorders.

Advantages and Disadvantages

The primary advantages of autologous marrow are that it is extensively available and that it lacks the immunologic complications of allogeneic marrow transplants, i.e., rejection or graft-vs-host disease. Since these problems do not exist with autologous marrow transplants, toxicity is limited mainly to that produced by the conditioning regimen. Potential disadvantages include the delayed marrow recovery (presumably due to previous damage to the hematopoietic stem cell compartment from cytotoxic therapy or, rarely, a flawed cryopreservation process) and the absence of the "graft-vs-leukemia" effect.

As discussed above, a more important disadvantage of autologous marrow transplants as currently practiced is the requirement for a normal (or nearly-normal) marrow at the time of harvest. This requirement excludes most patients with multiple myeloma, chronic lymphocytic leukemia and certain non-Hodgkin's lymphomas who would be very good candidates for intensive therapies using autologous marrow rescue. Moreover, even with apparent marrow remission, in some patients there exists the possibility of re-infusing occult malignant clonogenic cells, especially in those patients with pre-existing marrow involvement. It must be assumed that such cells could result in relapse after otherwise curative therapy. In addition, with certain cases of acute myelogenous leukemia there may be an intrinsic change in the stem cell that persists despite normal morphology, as well as normal immunophenotypic, clonogenic and karyotypic assays. In such cases, autologous marrow transplantation would presumably be doomed to failure, since no intrinsically normal stem cell population would exist.

Causes of Relapse after Autologous Marrow Transplantation

Paradoxically, the diseases most responsive to escalated-dose therapy (the hematologic malignancies) are also the diseases most likely to have marrow contamination with malignant cells. (To a lesser extent, this statement also applies to solid malignancies such as small-cell lung and breast cancer.) However, it must be emphasized that the most likely cause of recurrence following autologous marrow transplantation is failure of the conditioning regimen. This observation is derived from experience with syngeneic marrow transplants, where relapse rates are high even with leukemias in early remission but much more so with advanced disease. Therefore, the purging of malignant stem cells from the autologous marrow, although likely important in certain diseases, is clearly futile if effective conditioning regimens do not exist.

Selective Depletion (purging) of Malignant Cells

Contrary to what intuition suggests, the routine need for marrow purging, even in diseases that involve the marrow, is unproven. For instance, Burnett et al. gave acute myelogenous leukemia patients in first remission consolidation therapy consisting of intensive chemoradiotherapy and unpurged autologous marrow transplantation; long-term relapse-free survival was observed in a surprising number of these cases. Although these results have been discounted and ascribed to patient selection, they remain auspicious.

Nevertheless, at least for diseases characterized by marrow involvement, some selective depletion of malignant clonogenic cells ("purging") is probably required. Successful purging may depend on the degree of disparity between the malignant and normal hematopoietic stem cells. With diseases in which the malignant cell is closely related to the normal hematopoietic stem cell, as with the myeloid leukemias, purging may be more difficult than in diseases where malignant cells are less closely related to these stem cells, i.e., in the lymphoid malignancies.

Many methods of marrow purging have been tried; certain basic techniques are indicated in Table 5. Currently, a primary problem with purging is the current inability to reliably assay either normal or malignant hematopoietic stem cells. Therefore, the optimal method of purging remains uncertain, and may well be different for different diseases. Initially, physical methods such as density gradient separation were evaluated and found unsuccessful. More recently, the use of the monoclonal antibody technology (combined with a method of removing cells – such as using complement, a toxin or magnetic beads) or chemoseparation with a variety of chemotherapy agents (notably water – soluble congeners of cyclophosphamide, such as 4-hydroperoxycyclophosphamide [4-HC], mafosfamide [ASTA-Z]) have been the most popular. Many other methods are being developed, but none are standard approaches for any single disease – or likely to be applicable to all diseases. On the other hand, a method of positive, selection of hematopoietic stem cells would be very attractive, mainly by its widespread applicability. Such a goal is being pursued by many laboratories.

Choosing Autologous Rather than Allogeneic Marrow

Although autologous marrow transplants are most often considered in the context of patients without histocompatible donors, there are circumstances in which using autologous marrow may actually be preferable to using allogeneic marrow. In particular, the opportunity to avoid GVHD makes autologous more desirable than allogeneic marrow transplantation in a situation in which marrow contamination with malignant cells is unlikely (or when there is confidence in the efficacy of purging) and there is no evidence of an immunologic antitumor effect ("graft-vs-leukemia" or something similar) with the allogeneic marrow transplant. Currently this situation is probably present with some cases of Hodgkin's disease

Table 5. Marrow Purging Techniques for Autologous Marrow Transplantation

Technique	Examples
Physical	Density gradients
Immunologic	mostly using monoclonal antibodies + complement + toxins + magnetic beads
Pharmacologic	4-HC/ASTA-Z VP16-213 Doxorubicin Bleomycin Corticosteroids Vincristine Etc.

and certain malignant lymphomas. In these diseases, marrow involvement is relatively infrequent, especially during the early phases. Moreover, a "graft-vs-lymphoma" effect is undefined. Although it is more controversial, and depends on the results of ongoing studies with autologous marrow transplantation, the case of older (50–60 years of age) acute leukemia patients may eventually also be considered in this category. Finally, for those diseases in which the probability of cure is low with current conditioning regimens (e.g., most solid malignancies), the risks of allogeneic marrow transplantation are not justified. Autologous marrow transplants have been used almost exclusively in such clinical trials.

Patient Selection for Autologous Marrow Transplantation

Given the above considerations, which patients should be evaluated for autologous marrow transplantation? Patients with malignancies now considered curable using current conditioning regimens and syngeneic marrow transplants but who do not have suitable donors are probably the best candidates for autologous marrow transplantation. Such patients should also have a marrow in histologic remission at the time of harvest.

Although this recommendation is controversial, autologous marrow transplantation may be the treatment of choice for certain Hodgkin's disease and non-Hodgkin's lymphoma patients, i.e., those who have failed primary chemotherapy. Other disease categories are suitable for clinical research studies.

Peripheral Blood Stem-Cell Transplants

There are some patients who would be candidates for autologous marrow transplantation but in whom marrow cannot be easily harvested, e.g., those with extensive radiotherapy to the pelvis. In these patients cytapheresis and subsequent peripheral blood autologous stem cell transplants may be carried out, using roughly 10^{11} nucleated cells. Such grafts have successfully reconstituted hematopoiesis following myeloablative therapy.

Perhaps of even greater interest, the use of peripheral-blood autologous transplants may avoid heavy contamination of the circulating stem-cell component with tumor cells. This is probably best illustrated by circumstances in which marrow involvement is much more prominent than blood involvement, i.e., by non-leukemic disorders. Autologous peripheral-blood transplants are experimental.

Evaluation for Autologous Marrow Transplantation

Except for considerations of cell support, histocompatibility resting is not routinely required if the decision has been made to proceed with an autologous marrow transplant. However, a recent (i.e. within two weeks or so) bone marrow aspirate and biopsy is required both to document histologic marrow normalcy and to ensure that the marrow can be aspirated easily. More sophisticated studies to document the normalcy of the marrow may achieve importance in the future but are not routinely required at present.

Unrelated Donors for Transplantation

The use of volunteer unrelated donors is an area of intense clinical research interest. This interest is due to:

1. The favorable results of histocompatible allogeneic marrow transplantation in general;
2. The requirement for a greater number of suitable donors;
3. The feasibility of unrelated donors as suggested by preclinical and more limited clinical evidence;
4. The safety of marrow donation;
5. The current limitations of the alternative sources of marrow, i.e., autologous marrow (marrow remission or occult tumor cell contamination) and HLA partially-matched related donors (increased rejection or GVHD).

However, in order to have enough phenotypic-matched volunteer donors to reliably support this need, a very large registry of several hundred thousand volunteer donors will be required. Such registries may be initiated from existing apheresis banks without extraordinary resources, but they will be expensive to further develop and maintain. However, if slightly lesser degrees of matching were satisfactory (i.e., incompatibility at a single Class I or Class II alleles), much smaller registries would be required.

Since a high incidence of transplant-related complications occurs even with HLA-matched related donor transplants, it is possible that a greater incidence of severe complications would result from phenotypic-matched unrelated donor grafts. This would almost certainly be the case if donors less compatible were used. Therefore, such transplants may require improved methods of preventing or treating rejection or graft-vs-host disease to become clinically feasible. In any case, while it is possible and quite likely that the overall results of even phenotypic-matched unrelated marrow transplants will be somewhat inferior to genotypic-matched sibling transplants, the results will have to be roughly similar to justify the expense of these registries.

Finally, using unrelated donors opens the door to moral, legal and financial questions not posed with related donors. While unrelated volunteer donors cannot currently be regarded as a routine source of marrow for transplantation, their use might considered in certain high-priority younger patients, preferably by a center with a research interest in unrelated donor marrow transplantation.

Cell Support Considerations

Overview

Certain problems, such as severe pre-transplant allosensitization or any unusual blood type, require special consideration from apheresis units and blood banks. In addition, patients who receive marrow transplants from donors with incompatible major red blood cell groups require special manipulations to avoid hemolysis with the marrow reinfusion and in the immediate post-transplant period (see III, 3).

Allosensitization

A most difficult problem is that of severe allosensitization which may preclude the effective platelet transfusion that is required until the transplant is functional. Patients who are allosensitized to a lesser degree, but who do not have a sufficient number of donors due to an uncommon HLA type, may be equally difficult to support. (These patients are also unlikely to receive benefit from granulocyte transfusions, a modality now infrequently used.) While anecdotal experience suggests that epsilon aminocaproic acid (EACA, Amicar) might be used to diminish thrombocytopenic hemorrhage in such patients, a high risk of such hemorrhage remains. Therefore, transplantation should be undertaken only with trepidation if severe allosensitization to the best available platelet sources.

Erythrocyte Support Problems

The need to support patients with unusual red cell antigens is not unique to marrow transplantation. Given adequate notice, blood banking facilities can usually deal with these problems, often by stockpiling a supply of frozen blood.

ABO-incompatible Marrow Transplants

The problem with ABO- (or less likely, Rh-)incompatible marrow transfusion relates primarily to hemolysis, as there is little firm evidence that even major incompatibilities adversely affect engraftment, GVHD or survival. The special precautions required in patients who receive major red cell antigen (usually ABO) incompatible marrow include preventing hemolysis with the procedure and providing appropriate changes in transfusion support post-transplant. Several methods to overcome hemolysis have been employed, including plasmapheresis, the use of immunoabsorbent columns to decrease the isohemmagglutinin titer, and appropriate separation of the incompatible erythrocytes from donor marrow *ex vivo* by centrifugation. The problem with post-transplant transfusion supporting can be managed by selecting blood components that avoid incompatible red cells and plasma.

For both problems, consultation with the blood blank or apheresis staff during the planning stage of transplantation is recommended.

Organ Toxicity Screening

(Preliminary discussion of this topic was included in 3.5.2 and 3.5.4 above.) Patients should not have impairment of any organ system that would preclude an otherwise successful transplant. It is important to emphasize that pre-transplant impairment may be subclinical, only to become manifest after the "stress" of the conditioning regimen or transplant. Therefore, a systematic evaluations of the functioning of the liver, kidney, lungs, heart and perhaps certain endocrine glands should be performed. The history and physical examination of the patient are important, especially regarding prior therapy and serious co-morbid conditions that may produce a compromised organ, e.g., extensive anthracycline therapy and cardiac disease. In addition to routine hepatic and renal serum assays, a creatinine clearance, a full battery of pulmonary function tests and an assay of cardiac left ventricular function is desirable. While these tests may not reliably detect subclinical dysfunction, positive information may be helpful regarding various therapeutic components. For example, TBI may be avoided in a patient with even an increased risk factor for subsequent interstitial pneumonitis.

In male patients, it is also important to offer a semen analysis with the possibility of sperm banking. However, many men with malignant diseases who have undergone extensive cytotoxic chemotherapy will not have viable sperm.

Management of Existing Infections and Evaluation of Infection Potential

Pre-transplantation

Active pre-transplant infections

Patients with active or inadequately treated infections should be identified and started on appropriate therapy. While such infections should be resolved before the conditioning regimen begins, there are instances in which infections cannot be expected to improve without a successful graft. Pateints with severe neutropenia due to an otherwise untreatable underlying disease such as severe aplastic anemia, in which only successful marrow transplantation would increase the neutrophil count, are illustrative. In these cases marrow transplantation should not be delayed but rather expedited.

Reactivated host infections

It is also very important to be aware of previous infections that may be quiescent but which may be reactivated by the severe immunosuppression following the conditioning regimen. Examples include tuberculosis, aspergillosis and herpes viruses. At the very least, awareness, special precautions and perhaps prophylaxis may be indicated. In some cases such infections may actually contraindicate transplantation.

Donor infections

Similar considerations apply to donors. Although transmission of cytomegalovirus is presumed to be the most serious, transmission of other infections, such as malaria, human immunodeficiency virus and hepatitis B, have been reported.

Tumor Staging Studies

There are at least two reasons to document the activity of a malignant disease immediately before transplantation. First, active involvement (especially of a specific site such as the central nervous system) may be an indication for therapy additional to the conditioning regimen or perhaps for an altered conditioning regimen. Second, the presence of advanced disease is usually an important factor in the prognosis after marrow transplantation.

Since such evaluations are not generic to marrow transplantation (and will differ with various diseases), specific required studies will not be listed. In general, however, previous sites of disease should again be evaluated, as well as ones likely to be involved subclinically. Biopsy should be used without hesitation if findings would have a major influence on the decision to transplant or cause a major change in therapy.

Sperm Banking

Although many male patients may be sterile before conditioning, due to previous cytotoxic therapy. This option should be discussed. Regimens that contain total body irradiation are likely to be more sterilizing than those containing chemotherapy drugs alone. However, the potential of newer combination chemotherapy conditioning regimens (e.g. busulfan and cyclophosphamide) has not been evaluated in this regard.

Points of Emphasis

In many cases, preparation for transplantation is not urgent. In other circumstances, however, the need for prompt transplantation may compress the usual time required for preparation. In either situation, one must take particular care to ensure that the evaluation is meticulous, and that the patient and donor have had suitable time to arrive at a decision. The use of checklists and discussions with other staff on the Transplant Team to ensure completeness is often helpful. Also, it is most desirable that the refering physician be involved in the transplantation process, and especially that suitable follow-up is provided.

References

Appelbaum FR, Buckner CD (1986) Overview of the clinical relevance of autologous bone marrow transplantation. Clin Haematol 15: 1

Beatty PG, Clift RA, Mickelson EM, et al. (1985) Marrow transplantation from related donors other than HLA-identical siblings. N Engl J Med 313: 765

Bowden RA, Meyers JD (1985) Infectious complications following marrow transplantation. Plasma Ther Transfus Technol 6: 285

Bowden RA, Sayers M, Flournoy N, et al. (1986) Cytomegalovirus immune globulin and seronegative blood products to prevent primary cytomegalovirus infection after marrow transplantation. N Eng J Med 314: 1006

Burnett AK, Tansey P, Watkins R, et al. (1984) Transplantation of unpurged autologous bone marrow in acute myeloid leukemia in first remission. Lancet ii: 1068
Fefer A, Cheever MA, Greenberg PD (1983) Identical twin (syngeneic) marrow transplantation for hematologic malignancies. JNCI 76: 1269
Gale RP (1987) The role of bone marrow transplantation following nuclear accidents. Bone Marrow Transplantation 2: 1
Herzig GP (1981) Autologous marrow transplantation in cancer therapy. Prog Hematol 13: 1
Kessinger A, Armitage JD, Landmark JD, et al. (1986) Reconstitution of human hematopoietic function with autologous cryopreserved circulating stem cells. Exp Hematol 14: 192
Lasky LC, Warrentin PI, Kersfy JH, et al. (1983) Hemotherapy in patients undergoing blood group incompatible bone marrow transplantation. Transfusion 23: 277
McGlave P, Scott E, Ramsay N, et al. (1987) Unrelated donor bone marrow transplantation therapy for chronic myelogenous leukemia. Blood 70: 877
Vogelsang GB, Hess AD, Berkman AW, et al. (1985) An in vitro predictive test for graft-versus-host disease in patients with genotypic HLA-identical bone marrow transplants. N Engl J Med 313: 645

4. Who Pays?

As will become apparent below, bone marrow transplantation is a complex and expensive procedure. Estimates provided by different transplant centers range from $ 100,000 to $ 200,000. The cost will very much depend upon a patient's hospital course, since it is the hospitalization that accounts for a substantial fraction of the total bill. Who will pay for it? When marrow transplantation was first used in the early 70s', patient care funds were often provided by federal funding agencies in the form of grants to institutions carrying out marrow transplantation. Consequently, regardless of personal wealth or insurance coverage, a patient affected by a disease that could be approached via marrow transplantation could come to a center and be treated.

As more and more marrow transplants were carried out, and the success rate improved, less and less research funds oriented towards patient care were available. The procedure was no longer considered experimental and it was felt that insurance carriers should pay for it. Many insurance carriers, however, have continued to consider marrow transplantation an experimental procedure. Although certain indications, such as allogeneic marrow transplantation for the treatment of severe aplastic anemia or certain inherited disorders, is by now almost uniformly accepted as first line therapy, questions still arise in regards to other indications, for example marrow transplantation for the treatment of lymphoma.

This question is even more important in the context of autologous marrow transplantation. Although many investigators feel that for certain disease categories and patient groups, autologous marrow transplantation might offer the best prognosis, a true consensus has not been reached, and many insurance carriers have refused to pay for this procedure.

It will be important, therefore, for any patient in whom marrow transplantation, specifically autologous marrow transplantation is considered, to discuss these plans with their respective insurance company. It is usually helpful to have this information available at the time when a patient presents to a marrow transplant center. In any event, the billing office at the transplant center will always verify this information. Even if the procedure is covered it is possible that only 80% of the cost may be reimbursed. The remainder of the bill may be presented to the patient.

In the setting of allogeneic marrow transplantation, insurance carriers have usually been willing to pay for expenses incurred by the bone marrow donor, i.e. cost of short term hospitalization, anesthesia, time in the operating room, and brief post operative care. It should, however, also be noted that bone marrow donation will usually mean that the donor is away from his work at least for a few days, and possibly for several weeks if he is required to serve as a platelet transfusion donor after transplantation. It is helpful to discuss this with the donor's employer in order to avoid unpleasant surprises later on.

References

Kay HE, Lawler SD, Powles RL, Clink HM (1980) Cost of bone marrow transplants in acute myeloid leukaemia. The Lancet, I: 1067

Trigg ME (1986) The decision in pediatrics to go ahead with bone marrow transplant for a pediatric malignancy. Bone Marrow Transplantation 1: 111

Vaughan WP, Purtilo RB, Butler CD, Armitage JO (Editorial) (1986) Ethical and financial issues in autologous marrow transplantation: a symposium sponsored by the University of Nebraska Medical Center. Ann Int Med 105: 134

Watson JG, Clink HM, Powles RL, Jameson B, Kay HEM, Lumley H (1981) Acute myeloid leukaemia: comparison of support required during initial induction of remission and marrow transplantation in first remission. The Lancet, II: 957

III. Transplant Procedure

1. Donor Selection

Dependent upon the patient's disease, there may be one or more options when selecting a bone marrow donor. In contrast to most solid organ transplants a bone marrow transplant is generally from a related (family) donor, preferably identical with the patient for the major histocompatibility complex, HLA. However, the donor may also be a related HLA nonidentical family member, or in the rare instance when this is possible, a monozygotic (identical) twin. In recent years efforts have also been made to carry out transplants from volunteer unrelated donors (HLA identical or nonidentical) when no other alternatives exist, and finally, of course, the patient's own bone marrow (autologous) can be used (see II.3). In the latter case, we are not truly dealing with a *transplant* procedure, but rather the *reinfusion* of previously aspirated marrow. Table 6 illustrates which marrow source can be used in different disease categories. Table 7 lists and briefly defines potential marrow donors.

Table 6. Potential Marrow Sources for Different Disease Categories[a)]

- * Disease: Acquired, usually malignant diseases with intact hemopoietic stem cell function
  Potential Marrow Source:
  - Allogeneic
  - Syngeneic
  - Autologous
- * Disease: Acquired diseases affecting hemopoietic function
  Potential Marrow Source:
  - Allogeneic
  - Syngeneic
- * Disease: Congenital diseases
  Potential Marrow Source:
  - Allogeneic

a) excluding the possibility of xenogeneic marrow

When choosing a donor parameters other than histocompatibility also need to be taken into consideration (Table 8), and factors such as the potential donor's medical condition, the risks associated with anesthesia (during the marrow harvest), and psychological stability, including the donor's relationship to the pa-

Table 7. Potential Marrow Donors

* Autologous:	Patient's own marrow
* Syngeneic:	Monozygotic (identical) twin
* Allogeneic:	HLA genotypically identical sibling
	HLA phenotypically identical donor
	– Sibling
	– Parent
	– Other family member
	– Unrelated volunteer
	HLA nonidentical donor
	– Family member
	– Unrelated volunteer
* Xenogeneic:	Different species donor

Table 8. Factors Other than Histocompatibility Which Affect Donor Selection

ABO/Rh Blood Group	
Cytotoxic antibodies in patient serum	
Donor/Patient sex	
Donor pregnancy	
Donor age	
Viral Immunity	– Cytomegalovirus
	– Hepatitis virus
	– Human immunodeficiency virus

tient, may be relevant. Finally, patient age is of importance, since it appears that with syngeneic and autologous transplants a greater patient age is still compatible with survival compared to allogeneic transplants.

Since marrow aspiration is carried out on the anesthetized donor (general or spinal/epidural anesthesia), it is important to exclude the existence of any condition or illness that would increase the donor's anesthetic risk. This is of particular importance in female donors of child bearing age. If a female donor is being considered, a pregnancy test should be obtained. If a potential donor is found to be pregnant, ideally an alternative donor should be searched for. If no such alternative is available, the transplant may perhaps be delayed. In patients with certain diagnoses, i.e. chronic myelogenous leukemia, or acute nonlymphoblastic leukemia in first remission, such an approach may be feasible. In other instances, for instance advanced leukemia, this may not be possible. In such a situation, the potential risk to the pregnant woman and the fetus will have to be weighed against the potential benefit to the patient. This may be a very difficult ethical decision but in some instances pregnant women have served as marrow donors without any harm to the fetus.

Age is, similarly, a relative contraindication for marrow donation because of the known increase in anesthetic risk with increasing age. Most transplant centers have excluded individuals more than 60 years of age from marrow donation. In all instances, however, it is important to evaluate potential donors individually.

In a recent review of 3,290 marrow harvesting procedures, virtually all donors were found to experience pain at the marrow aspiration sites for a few days following the harvest. Only 9 donors (0.3%) had potentially life threatening complications, infectious or cardiovascular in nature, and all recovered uneventfully. However, this report also mentions one donor from another center (unpublished observations) who could not be resuscitated following a cardiac arrest during anesthesia.

Next to the patient's underlying disease the most important factor determining outcome after transplantation, at the present time, appears to be the degree of histocompatibility with the marrow donor. The major histocompatibility complex antigens, termed HLA (human leukocyte antigen), are coded for by genes located on the short arm of chromosome 6. In addition, there are so-called minor, or non-HLA histocompatibility antigens. It has been very difficult in man to identify minor antigens, and basically all transplants that have been carried out to date have dealt with donor and recipient pairs characterized for HLA, but not for other antigens. The inheritance of HLA genes follows a Mendelian pattern, i.e. every individual will have inherited one gene region, called a haplotype, from the father, and one from the mother. HLA antigens are highly polymorphic. By definition, however, there can be at most four haplotypes within each nuclear family (parents and children). Consequently, each patient who has a sibling has a theoretical chance of one in four that the sibling is HLA identical with the patient (unless a cross-over has occurred), and in fact 40% of caucasian patients who have siblings are found to have an HLA identical donor. HLA identity is determined by using serological and cellular assays. Present HLA terminology is based on agreements reached at the Nineth International Histocompatibility Workshop. Histocompatibility typing should be carried out by an experienced laboratory, which has access to the latest typing reagents and uses the internationally accepted terminology. Generally, such laboratories will type patient and potential donor cells for HLA A, B, C, and DR, and possibly also DQ and DP using alloantisera. In addition, cells will be set up against each other in a mixed leukocyte culture (MLC) to determine whether other antigens, not recognized by serological typing, lead to allogeneic stimulation of these cells as measured by radioactive thymidine uptake into replicating DNA. These antigens are referred to as HLA-D antigens. Occasionally patients and their siblings have been typed and found to be completely identical at least in appearance (phenotype) for all serologically determined antigens, yet the respective cells show mutual reactivity in mixed leukocyte culture. Such a discrepancy is observed in less than 5% of sibling typings. Furthermore, even if both serological typing and mixed leukocyte culture results show identity, it is still possible that this is due to phenotypic identity only (see Fig. 1B). This can occur, for example, if the parents each express the same antigens on one of their respective haplotypes as can occur with one of the very common haplotypes, i.e. in the caucasian population, HLA A2/B7. Thus, both the father and the mother may have HLA A2/B7 phenotypes, which are derived from different *genetic* backgrounds. Consequently, one of their children might have inherited the paternal A2/B7 haplotype, and one the maternal A2/B7 haplotype. Unless the parent typing is also available, a clear segregation of the genetic information cannot be determined, and occasionally it may not be possible to separate phenotypic from genotypic identity. Hence, whenever available, parents should be included in HLA typing studies. Occasionally typing of children may also be useful. The decision as to who else in the family should be typed must be arrived at after a discussion with an expert in an HLA laboratory, ideally at a bone marrow transplant facility.

Although most transplants carried out and reported to date have involved an HLA identical donor, the possibility of marrow transplantation should not be dismissed immediately if no HLA identical family member can be found. The number of HLA nonidentical transplants carried out at various centers is growing rapidly. Early results are encouraging, in that patients who were transplanted from a donor who differs for only one HLA antigen region (HLA A, or B, or D/DR) have a prognosis not significantly inferior to that observed with completely HLA identical transplants. This is particularly true if patients are being transplanted for a lymphohemopoietic malignancy while in chemotherapy-induced remission. Results are less good in patients transplanted while in relapse or for non-malignant conditions, such as severe aplastic anemia. Results are less encouraging as the extent of histocompatibility increases, i.e. as two or even three antigenic regions (complete haplotype) are mismatched between donor and recipient. Problems include an increased incidence and severity of graft-vs-host disease, failure of engraftment, and infectious complications, both early and late after transplantation.

Experience with unrelated volunteer marrow donors is still quite limited. A crucial limiting factor is the availability of a suitably matched donor. The chances of finding such a donor is better with "common" HLA phenotypes (examples are shown in Table 3) than with rare ones. Several successful transplants with phenotypically matched volunteer donors have been reported, but overall the success rate, even in patients who would be good risk candidates for HLA genotypically identical transplants, is low. More importantly, even patients who have successful engraftment appear to have severely delayed immunereconstitution and may conceivably never become completely immunocompetent.

In some instances these limitations do not apply. For example, in a child with severe combined immunedeficiency as pointed out earlier, haploidentical transplantation from father or mother, usually after T cell depletion of the marrow, can be carried out successfully. In this setting, engraftment is often incomplete, i.e. only T lymphocytes may engraft, but this is all that is required in order to render these children immunocompetent. They do well in regards to their own hemopoietic system and also B cells.

ABO incompatibility represents less of a problem in marrow transplantation than in renal transplantation. Blood group differences between donor and recipient may require manipulation of the marrow or isoagglutinin removal in the patient before marrow infusion (see III, 3). The effect of cytotoxic antibodies on marrow engraftment is still disputed. However, patients with cytotoxic antibodies have generally been treated with plasmapheresis pretransplant to remove antibodies.

There are data to suggest that sex differences may carry an increased risk of graft rejection in patients with aplastic anemia (M > F) or may cause more graft-vs-host disease (F > M). Similarly, prior pregnancy in female donors and increased donor age have been found to increase the probability of graft-vs-host disease in some studies. There has always been concern that viruses may be transmitted from the donor to the patient, who may then be at high risk of developing a symptomatic infection because of transplant-related immunosuppression. If there is a choice between a CMV^+ and a CMV^- donor (all other factors being identical), the CMV^- donor is thought to be preferable because the risk of CMV infection in the patient (particularly in the CMV^- patient) would be expected to be lower. This assessment has been challenged recently by the results of a study using T cell depleted marrow.

In addition to allogeneic transplantation, autologous marrow transplantation has been used, on an experimental basis, in an increasing number of patients. Although follow-up observation with autologous transplants to date is generally shorter than with allogeneic transplants, some autologous transplant results are encouraging. Since autologous transplantation circumvents transplant-related problems such as the development of GVHD, physicians may face the question of an autologous versus an allogeneic transplant if an HLA identical family donor is available. Such a decision will depend upon the patient's underlying disease, the disease stage, the patient's age and other medical conditions. If a patient is more than 50 years of age (at some centers more than 45 years) but otherwise would be considered a candidate for transplantation, autologous transplant might be the best available approach. Of course, if the patient has a disease involving hemopoietic stem cells such as aplastic anemia or chronic myelogenous leukemia (see Table 6), this is not an option. At present, it is generally accepted that a patient less than 45 or 50 years of age with an HLA identical marrow donor should have an allogeneic transplant.

If no HLA identical donor is available, the decision becomes more difficult. Results with allogeneic HLA nonidentical donors have been discussed already. Many questions remain unanswered with regards to autologous transplantation. When should one proceed with autologous transplantation? Should autologous transplantation with marrow purging be carried out? Is there a graft-vs-leukemia effect? One might expect this to occur in an allogeneic transplant where histocompatibility differences exist, but not in an autologous or a syngeneic transplant. Answers to these questions are not yet available and the decision regarding autologous transplantation at present depends upon the existence of investigational protocols at a given transplant center.

References

Bensinger WI, Buckner CD, Thomas ED, Clift RA (1982) ABO-incompatible marrow transplants. Transplantation 33: 427

Blazar BR, Lasky LC, Perentesis JP, Watson KV, Steinberg SE, Filipovich AH, Orr HT, Ramsay NKC (1986) Successful donor cell engraftment in a recipient of bone marrow from a cadaveric donor. Blood 67: 1655

Bone-marrow autotransplantation in man. (Report of an International Cooperative Study) (1986) The Lancet, II: 960

Bortin MM, Buckner CD (1983) Major complications of marrow harvesting for transplantation. Exp Hematol 11: 916

Bowden RA, Sayers M, Flournoy N, Newton B, Banaji M, Tho mas ED, Meyers JD (1986) Cytomegalovirus immune globulin and seronegative blood products to prevent primary cytomegalovirus infection after marrow transplantation. New Eng J Med 314: 1006

Braine HG, Sensenbrenner LL, Wright SK, Tutschka PJ, Saral R, Santos GW (1982) Bone marrow transplantation with major ABO blood group incompatibility using erythrocyte depletion of marrow prior to infusion. Blood 60: 420

Buckner CD, Clift RA, Sanders JE, Stewart P, Bensinger WI, Doney K, Sullivan KM, Witherspoon RP, Deeg HJ, Appelbaum FR, Storb R, Thomas ED (1984) Marrow harvesting from normal donors. Blood 64: 630

Duquesnoy RJ, Zeevi A, Marrari M, Hackbarth S, Camitta B, for the Milwaukee Children's Hospital Bone Marrow Transplantation Team (1983) Bone marrow transplantation for severe aplastic anemia using a phenotypically HLA-identical, SB-compatible unrelated donor. Transplantation 35: 566

Filipovich AH, Ramsay NKC, McGlave P, Quinones R, Winslow C, Heinitz KJ, Arthur D, Kersey JH (1983) Mismatched bone marrow transplantation at the university of Minnesota: Use of related donors other than HLA MLC identical siblings and T cell depletion. Recent Advances in Bone Marrow Transplantation R. P. Gale (ed.) Alan R. Liss, Inc., New York, pp 769

Fischer A, Durandy A, de Villartay JP, Vilmer E, Le Deist F, Gerota I, Griscelli C (1986) HLA-haploidentical bone marrow transplantation for severe combined immunodeficiency using E rosette fractionation and cyclosporine. Blood 67: 444

Gale RP (1986) Potential utilization of national HLA-typed donor pool for bone marrow transplantation. Transplantation 42: 54

Gingrich RD, Howe CWS, Goeken NE, Ginder GD, Kugler JW, Tewfik HH, Klassen LW, Armitage JO, Fyfe MA (1985) The use of partially matched, unrelated donors in clinical bone marrow transplantation. Transplantation 39: 526

Hansen JA, Clift RA, Thomas ED, Buckner CD, Storb R, Giblett ER (1980) Transplantation of marrow from an unrelated donor to a patient with acute leukemia. New Eng J Med 303: 565

Hows JM, Yin JL, Marsh J, Swirsky D, Jones L, Apperley JF, James DCO, Smithers S, Batchelor JR, Goldman JM, Gordon-Smith EC (1986) Histocompatible unrelated volunteer donors compared with HLA nonidentical family donors in marrow transplantation for aplastic anemia and leukemia. Blood 68: 1322

Lonnqvist B, Ringden O, Wahren B, Gahrton G, Lundgren G (1984) Cytomegalovirus infection associated with and preceding chronic graft-versus-host disease. Transplantation 38: 465

O'Reilly RJ (1987) Current developments in marrow transplantation. Transplant Proc 19: 92

Powles RL, Kay HEM, Clink HM, Barrett A, Depledge MH, Sloane J, Lumley H, Lawler SD, Morgenstern GR, McElwain TJ, Dady PJ, Jameson B, Watson JG, Leigh M, Hedley D, Filshie J, Robinson B (1983) Mismatched family donors for bone-marrow transplantation as treatment for acute leukaemia. The Lancet, I: 612

Storb R (1987) Critical issues in bone marrow transplantation. Transplant Proc 19: 2774

2. Conditioning Regimens

General Considerations

Immediately before marrow transplantation, patients are generally given a course of intensive chemoradiotherapy (including total body irradiation) or, alternatively, chemotherapy alone. This treatment is known as the conditioning (or preparative) regimen and varies in composition according to the disease being treated and the type of marrow used for transplantation. The function of conditioning is two-fold – i.e., immunosuppression and/or removal of unwanted cell populations, as discussed more fully in II.3.

A list of agents frequently used in current conditioning regimens is presented in Table 9. These agents are listed according to their putative primary function, as certain agents (even when used in very high doses) tend to have predominantly either immunosuppressive or antineoplastic qualities. Some – e.g., total body irradiation (TBI) – have both. In the circumstance of allogeneic marrow transplantation for hematologic malignancies, agents with potent immunosuppressive and antineoplastic features are required. However, it is neither necessary nor always desirable to use components with both properties. For instance, antineoplastic effects are undesirable in non-malignant disorders, whereas immunosuppression is not required in syngeneic or autologous marrow transplantation. (Some cases of syngeneic marrow transplantation for aplastic anemia may be an exception.) Antithymocyte globulin (ATG), and cyclophosphamide are examples of agents used primarily for their immunosuppressive features, while busulfan

Table 9. Conditioning Regimen Components

Agents Used Primarily for Immunosuppression
- Anti-thymocyte gloculin
- Cyclophosphamide
- Total lymphoid irradiation (TLI)

Agents Used Primarily for Antineoplastic Effects
- Busulfan/Dimethylmyleran
- Carmustine
- Cytarabine
- Etoposide/Tenoposide

Agents Used for Both Purposes
- Total body irradiation (TBI)
- Melphalan

and carmustine are examples of agents used primarily for their antineoplastic effects. However, such a separation of function for these components is undoubtedly an oversimplification; e.g., cyclophosphamide is an active antineoplastic agent for certain malignancies, and busulfan has immunosuppressive effects at the doses used in conditioning regimens.

Single-agent therapy is not widely used for conditioning, save for previously untransfused aplastic anemia patients in which cyclophosphamide 200 mg/kg is standard therapy. Multiple agents are used because tolerable doses of most single agents (other than TBI or perhaps melphalan) provide only marginal immunosuppression in other circumstances, and additional agents are required. Multiple agents are also are deemed necessary for satisfactory antineoplastic effects. These considerations have led to the construction of two-agent regimens such as cyclophosphamide plus TBI (CY + TBI) and cyclophosphamide plus busulfan (BUCY) for marrow transplant conditioning (examples of each are detailed in Tables 10 and 11). Such regimens provide satisfactory immunosuppression for histocompatible allogeneic grafts, and acceptable antineoplastic effects, providing they are used for the hematologic malignancies in an early (preferably first) remission or stable phase. As with other antineoplastic therapies, relapse rates generally rise dramatically with more advanced disease.

While a further increase in the number of antileukemic agents might enhance antitumor effects, this approach has proven difficult, primarily because current conditioning regimes have a marginal therapeutic index that would probably decrease with the addition of more agents. Especially in allogeneic marrow transplantation, even a slight degree of additional toxicity might produce an unacceptable increase in overall toxicity that might negate improved antitumor effects. As discussed below, however, this theoretical limitation should not be regarded as absolute.

Detailed Requirements of the Conditioning Regimen

Immunosuppression

In allogeneic marrow transplants, immunosuppression of the host-vs-graft reaction is usually required for stable engraftment. (The concept of providing "space" or "niches" for the stem cells to relocate and proliferate is presumably encompassed in this function as well.) Certain congenital immunodeficiency syndromes (e.g., severe combined immunodeficiency disease, SCID) are the exceptions to this rule, as the intrinsic immunosuppression of SCID abrogates this requirement. Also, immunosuppression is not required in syngeneic or autologous marrow transplants.

The immunosuppression required for a successful allogeneic marrow transplant depends on several potentially interrelated factors. These include the degree of histocompatibility, the degree of underlying immunosuppression of the primary disease and its therapy, sensitization via previous exposure to allogeneic cells or tissueres (especially via blood transfusions), and the number and type of marrow cells infused.

Histocompatibility. Experimentally, progressive degrees of histoincompatibility require more immunosuppression for sustained engraftment; more limited human data confirm this funding. While current conditioning regimens for leukemia that precede histocompatible marrow transplantation are usually sufficiently immunosuppressive to prevent graft rejection, preliminary evidence in histoincompatible marrow transplantation indicates that currently used conditioning regimens are not optimal, and that modifications likely will be required to produce reliable engraftment for these transplants. Aplastic anemia is a somewhat different situation, since the additional immunosuppression offered by antineoplastic components such as total body irradiation is often lacking, and graft rejection is a problem in aplastic anemia, chiefly in those previously-transfused patients who received cyclophosphamide (200 mg/kg) conditioning alone. The use of similar conditioning in untransfused patients or the use of cyclophosphamide plus a second immunosuppressive modality – e.g., total lymphoid irradiation – or, alternatively, buffy-coat transfusions in previously-transfused patients reduces the risk of rejection.

Underlying disease. In diseases other than those with severe intrinsic immunodeficiency, the degree of immunosuppression is more variable and potent immunosuppression via conditioning is deemed necessary to produce stable engraftment. Nevertheless, it is likely that in certain diseases (e.g., Hodgkin's disease) the immunosuppression produced by the basic disease as well as that contributed by conventional therapy is probably such that less immunosuppression is required from the conditioning regimen. Whether this postulate could or should be exploited clinically is another matter, but theoretically this situation might allow an increase in the antineoplastic effects of conditioning elements, concomitant with a decrease in the immunosuppressive ones, without additional toxicity.

Sensitization. Blood transfusions given before transplantation sensitize patients against non-HLA histocompatibility determinants, and a previous history of blood transfusions is the chief prognostic factor in patients with severe aplastic anemia who reject HLA-identical transplants following cyclophosphamide conditioning. For hematologic malignancies, however, additional antineoplastic therapy often involves TBI, usually given in doses of 500–1,000 cGy (unfractionated) to 1,200–1,575 cGy (fractionated). Such therapy concomitantly produces such profound immunosuppression that graft rejection is rare among leukemic patients who receive unmanipulated HLA-identical marrow transplants. Lesser data suggest that intensive combination chemotherapy conditioning functions adequately in this regard as well.

Composition of the graft. The composition of the marrow graft is undoubtedly an important determinant for the achievement of stable engraftment. Currently, however, it is difficult to quantify the composition (in man) of hematopoietic stem and accessory cells, due primarily to a lack of suitable assays. For instance, the "minimum engrafting dose" of hematopoietic stem cells in man is likely variable depending on the factors noted above and is a small multiple of 10^8/kg of patient body weight. Marrow nucleated cell doses below 3×10^8/kg of body weight have been observed to be a negative prognostic sign for engraftment in transfused aplastic anemia patients conditioned with cyclophosphamide before histocompatible marrow transplants. While it is likely that the minimum engrafting dose is less with syngeneic transplants, this observation is of limited clinical significance, since such amounts of marrow can usually be taken from healthy donoers without difficulty. The role of accessory cells in re-establishing stable hematopoiesis is not clear, although it has been observed that selectively removing T-lymphocytes from the marrow to abrogate graft-vs-host disease increases the risk of graft rejection, presumably because of this mechanism (see IV.3). To overcome this effect, additional immunosuppression is likely required. Moreover, when several factors are combined, stable engraftment may be a very difficult problem; for instance, with current conditioning regimes T-cell depletion in histoincompatible grafts is associated with a high rate of graft failure.

There are several ways to approach this area. Obviously, histoincompatible grafts should only be used in special situations, and transfusions (especially from family members) should be avoided whenever possible. However, it is likely that most transplant centers currently employ these measures, and more effective conditioning is required for the other circumstances noted. As noted previously, merely increasing the dose of existing cytotoxins may produce immunosuppressive effects but produce no change in survival due to increased toxicity. For example, adding TBI to cyclophosphamide as conditioning for allogeneic marrow transplantation for aplastic anemia clearly reduces the risk of rejection, but at the expense of increasing the rate of fatal interstitial pneumonitis. Agents other than those used for antineoplastic effects (e.g., TBI) are probably optimal; donor buffy-coat infusions post-transplantation, antithymocyte globulin, total lymphoid irradiation and certain monoclonal antibody complexes are examples.

Ablation of Unwanted Cell Populations

When an abnormal cell population is present, the conditioning regimen is primarily (and often solely) responsible for its removal. Usually the unwanted cell population is malignant; the majority of marrow transplant patients have had hematologic malignancies, mostly leukemias. There is no intrinsic reason, however, that malignancies that do not involve the marrow (i.e., some malignant lymphomas and non-hematologic cancers) cannot be successfully treated with marrow transplantation regimens. In this circumstance, the transplant is purely a "rescue" device for ablative-dose cytotoxic therapy, rather than serving this function plus replacing a diseased organ (as might be more appropriate for a leukemia). In other instances the removal of a non-malignant cell population may be necessary – e.g., in patients with thalassemia major. There even may be circumstances in which a normal (in a qualitative sense) cell population must be ablated (e.g., in some cases of aplastic anemia).

The ablation of unwanted cell populations poses a major challenge to successful marrow transplantation, a fact underscored by the high recurrence rates (usually but not always of host origin) that currently plague the use of marrow transplantation for malignancy. Over the past decade, the use of "early" transplantation (i.e., generally in the first or stable phase) has been the chief method for decreasing recurrence rates. Transplantation relatively early in the course of a malignant disease produces a more favorable result than transplantation delayed until end-stage malignancy is present, presumably because it is difficult to eradicate highly resistant tumor stem cells inherently present in advanced malignancy. In addition, patients with an end-stage malignant disease are often heavily pretreated and have resultant organ dysfunction (clinical or subclinical) that may increase post-transplant toxicity. For example, marrow transplantation performed early (usually during first or second remission) in the course of a malignancy "sensitive" to cytotoxic therapy, such as acute leukemia, produces much better cure rates than when performed during advanced relapse. However, even in the cases of acute leukemias transplanted in first remission, or chronic myelogenous leukemia in stable phase using histocompatible marrow, recurrence rates of 20–40% have been observed. In these diseases, situations other than first complete remission or stable phase are associated with higher recurrence rates. Moreover, failures due to inadequate tumor ablation are especially common in non-hematologic malignant diseases transplanted at any stage. As discussed previously, simple augmentations of current conditioning regimens have generally not altered this situation, reflecting both the intrinsic resistance of malignant cell populations and the marginal therapeutic index of these regimens.

One might think, therefore, that marrow transplantation perhaps should be limited to patients in first remission. However, there are problems with this approach. First, marrow transplant regimens are currently, and are likely to be for the foreseeable future, more toxic (and expensive) than even intensive conventional therapy. Thus, marrow regimens are indicated primarily when conventional regimens are unlikeley to produce durable remissions. As primary therapy improves, it will become more difficult to justify marrow transplantation in first remission unless high-risk subgroups can be identified, and marrow transplant regimens may be more appropriately used as salvage therapy. There is a frequently-overlooked problem with this approach, namely that the residue of patients who fail these improved primary therapy regimens will be much more refractory to existing conditioning regimens, producing an apparent decrease in the efficacy of such therapies. Therefore, if primary conventional treatment regimens improve markedly, marrow transplant regimens will need to be used promptly at the first sign of failure, as well as to attain greater efficacy to be useful.

Major Conditioning Regimens in Current Use

The following sections briefly detail the rationale, the results, and general administration of several currently used regimens. It is not intended as a substitute for scrutiny of the original reports.

Cyclophosphamide

In untransfused patients with aplastic anemia, cyclophosphamide in an intravenous dose of 50 mg/kg daily × 4 days (total dose = 200 mg/kg) produces stable engraftment with a low rate of rejection. In addition, there are data suggesting that somewhat lower doses may be as efficacious. Cyclophosphamide, either alone or in combination, is given with the following precautions:

Patient selection. Patients with pre-existing cardiac disease and those with abnormal urinary function, especially obstructive uropathy, should be considered for alternative therapy. The former is discussed below; the latter is important since good renal and urologic function is required to excrete the toxic metabolite acrolein, which produces excessive uroepithelial damage unless diluted and excreted promptly.

Hydration. Suitable hydration is vital to minimize severe hemorrhagic cystitis; cyclophosphamide has an antidiuretic hormone (ADH)-like effect on the kidney that complicates this requirement. Hyperhydration at 3,000 ml/m^2/day with a crystalloid intravenous solution should be initiated before cyclophosphamide is given to establish good urine flow, and should be continued for 48 hours after the last dose. Prophylactic diuretics such as furosemide (20 mg intravenously) are given immediately after cyclophosphamide, and as needed to keep a urine output of more than 100 ml per hour. Additional furosemide is used as needed to keep the morning body weight within 1–2 kg of baseline. Alternatively, the uroprotectant 2-mercaptoethane sulphonate (Mesna) can be used without this degree of hyperhydration.

Cardiotoxicity avoidance. The cardiomyopathy associated with cyclophosphamide is highly lethal and is usually observed with doses of 200 mg/kg or greater. Due to the devastating consequences of this rare complication, it is reasonable to assume that cardiac compromise of any etiology may predispose to the severe hemorrhagic myopericarditis occasionally seen with high-dose cyclophosphamide, although this is in fact unproven, as cardiomyopathy certainly occurs in patients without a prior history of cardiac disease.

There is little evidence that patients can be successfully treated once this complication arises. Giving the proper dose of cyclophosphamide is probably the most important preventive measure. Many centers use calculations based on ideal body weight. Alternatively, body surface area may be used to calculate the dose of cyclophosphamide.

Cyclophosphamide Plus Total Body Irradiation (TBI)

The pioneering efforts of Dr. E. D. Thomas and his colleagues in the field of allogeneic marrow transplantation for hematologic malignancy have proved the efficacy of the intensive chemoradiotherapy regimen cyclophosphamide plus TBI. In theory, TBI has unique benefits, especially in the treatment of leukemia –

namely, the lack of cross-resistance to chemotherapeutic drugs, the ability to treat pharmacologic sanctuaries and the potent immunosuppression required for allogeneic marrow transplantation. While additional benefits of cyclophosphamide are assumed rather than proven, the non-hématologic toxicity spectrum of cyclophosphamide is different from TBI, so these agents probably do not produce serious additive toxicity when used together. Also, cyclophosphamide has been shown to possess antitumor activity as a single agent in doses used in transplantation. In any case, cyclophosphamide (90–200 mg/kg) plus TBI (500–1,000 cGy in a single dose or 1,200–1,575 cGy in a fractionated schedule), usually but not invariably in the sequence of drug before radiotherapy, has become a standard conditioning regimen for hematologic malignancy.

When used with histocompatible marrow transplantation in acute leukemia in first remission, or chronic myelogenous leukemia in initial stable (or chronic) phase, relapse rates following cyclophosphamide plus TBI conditioning regimens are usually around 25%. However, when patients are transplanted in situations of more advanced leukemia (i.e., initial failure to achieve remission, initial relapse, second or subsequent remission or resistant relapse of acute leukemia, or accelerated or blast phase of chronic myelogenous leukemia), relapse rates rise to nearly 50% or even more. Therefore, while it may be argued that cyclophosphamide plus TBI represents an adequate antileukemic regimen for selected leukemic patients (i.e., those in remission or early stable phase), more effective tactics will be required to increase cure rates in patients with leukemia advanced beyond initial remission or stable phase. Moreover, it is not clear that cyclophosphamide plus TBI is optimal for other hematologic malignancies, and it is even more unlikely that this regimen is suitable for most non-hematologic malignancies. Specifically, most solid tumors are not very responsive to high-dose cyclophosphamide and often are much less radiosensitive than hematologic cancers.

With doses of TBI in excess of 1,000 cGy, permanent marrow ablation is usually assumed but is probably not universal. On the other hand, the non-hematologic toxicity of cyclophosphamide plus TBI is severe but largely reversible. Minor reversible complications are frequent and include nausea, emesis, alopecia, transient skin rash and abnormal liver functioning. More serious side effects include hemorrhagic cystitis and cardiomyopathy, veno-occlusive disease of the liver and interstitial pneumonitis.

It must be emphasized, however, that while "cyclophosphamide plus TBI" is often referred to as a uniform regimen, this is in fact not the case; three examples of this regimen in use are listed in Table 10. Specifically, cyclophosphamide is usually given for 2 days at 60 mg/kg daily several days before TBI, but has been given in other doses, e.g., 50 mg/kg daily for 3 or 4 days. Moreover, the cyclophosphamide dose has been calculated by both actual and ideal body weight, and has been given both before and after TBI. TBI has been administered even more variably; it is unlikely that any two institutions use TBI in exactly the same manner. Some regimens use single-fraction TBI, 500–1,000 cGy, while others use fractionated TBI, 1,200–1,575 cGy. In addition to the variables of total dose and fractionation, a bewildering variety of sources and dose-rates have been used. This heterogeneity precludes a simple evaluation of regimens of cyclo-

Table 10. Cyclophosphamide plus TBI Regimens in Common Use

Agent	Daily Dose	Schedule	Total Dose
A.			
Cyclophosphamide	60 mg/kg	Daily × 2 (days -5, -4)	120 mg/kg
Fractionated TBI	200 cGy (×2)	Twice daily × 3 (days -3, -2, -1)	1,200 cGy
B.			
Cyclophosphamide	60 mg/kg	Daily × 2 (days -8, -7)	120 mg/kg
Fractionated TBI	200 cGy	Daily × 6 (days -6, -5, -4, -3, -2, -1)	1,200 cGy
C.			
Cyclophosphamide	50 mg/kg	Daily × 4 (days -8, -7, -6, -5)	200 mg/kg
Fractionated TBI	300 cGy	Daily × 4 (days -4, -3, -2, -1)	1,200* cGy

* Lung shielding after 900 cGy

phosphamide 60 mg/kg daily × 2 plus TBI, and prevents the identification of a superior regimen. However, a prospectively randomized study in Seattle revealed a modest superiority of cyclophosphamide plus fractionated TBI 1,200 cGy versus single-fraction TBI 1,000 cGy.

Three commonly used dose-schedules are indicated in Table 10, and include cyclophosphamide 60 mg/kg daily × 2 followed by fractionated TBI 200 cGy twice daily × 3 days (denoted as A) or once daily × 6 days (denoted as B), or cyclophosphamide 200 mg/kg followed by daily fractionated TBI 300 cGy × 4, with lung shielding for the third dose (denoted as C). Bone marrow is usually infused 0–24 hours after the TBI. Certain other modifications of this regimen are discussed below.

Variants of Cyclophosphamide Plus TBI

Cyclophosphamide plus total lymphoid irradiation (TLI). When radiotherapy is given for its immunosuppressive rather than its antineoplastic effects, it is neither necessary nor desirable to irradiate the whole body. Specifically, toxicity to such radiosensitive organs as the lungs can be avoided to theoretically improve the therapeutic index of the conditioning. Based on preclinical data, the use of wide-field radiotherapy to lymphatic regions is profoundly immunosuppressive, and is less toxic than corresponding doses of TBI. Accordingly, TLI given in single doses of 300–750 cGy or fractionated doses in the range of 1,200 cGy, have been substituted for TBI in patients with severe aplastic anemia at high risk for graft rejection following allogeneic marrow transplantation. Such doses of TLI can also be given for additional immunosuppression with TBI regimens used to eradicate hematologic malignancy. This is probably most useful with histoincompatible transplants and/or T-cell depletion of the marrow.

Radiochemotherapy. The order of agents has been reversed, with hyperfraction of the TBI to 1,320 cGy in 11 (120 cGy) fractions (11 × 120 = 1,320) before cyclophosphamide 120 mg/kg (2 × 60 = 120 mg/kg). Lung shielding and boost electron therapy to the underlying ribs are also features of this regimen. Preliminary data suggests this regimen is at least no worse, and perhaps better, in its antileukemic effects than the parent regimen, especially in a group of second remission acute lymphocytic leukemia (ALL) patients.

Drug substitutions or additions. It would be difficult, within the scope of this Chapter to include most of the regimens with drug substitutions or additional agents added. However, several of the more common ones will be discussed briefly below.

Cytarabine in conventional dose (e.g., 100 mg/m^2 by continuous infusion daily × 5 days) or in high dose (i.e., 3 gm/m^2 twice daily × 6 days) has been used in leukemias before TBI. Conventional dose cytarabine plus cyclophosphamide (120 mg/kg) and single-fraction TBI (500 cGy) has been found useful in chronic myelogenous leukemia in an initial stable phase. The high-dose (i.e., 3 gm/m^2) regimen (without cyclophosphamide) has been used in acute lymphoblastic leukemia in second remission with fractionated TBI (1,200 cGy) with a suggestion of improved results compared to the parent regimen. Etoposide (i.e., 60 mg/kg × 1) has been used after the 1,320 cGy hyperfractionated TBI regimen mentioned above in high-risk acute leukemia with encouraging preliminary results. Melphalan (180 mg/m^2) has been used in a similar fashion.

Busulfan Plus Cyclophosphamide

This regimen was developed by Dr. G. W. Santos and colleagues to treat acute myelogenous leukemia. It was designed to avoid the use of TBI, which replaced with busulfan. Since TBI is avoided, this regimen may be administered at different institutions in a much more consistent fashion than cyclophosphamide plus TBI. In the parent regimen, busulfan 1 mg/kg is given orally every 6 hours × 16 doses (total dose 16 mg/kg of ideal body weight) followed by cyclophosphamide 50 mg/kg IV daily × 4 (= 200 mg/kg). Tuschka, et al., have used the same busulfan dose with a lower dose of cyclophosphamide, i.e., 60 mg/kg × 2 (= 120 mg/kg), and reported, in a preliminary study, at least equivalent results. In addition, lower doses of busulfan with cyclophosphamide have been used in conditioning regimens for non-malignant disease such as thalassemia major. In contrast to cyclophosphamide plus TBI, immediate side effects (specifically nausea and emesis, skin changes) are less common. The serious toxicity of busulfan plus cyclophosphamide tends to be hepatic (veno-occlusive disease). Generalized seizures also have been oberved in some cases in which prophylactic phenytoin has not been used. Interestingly, the rate of ablation of existing marrow function is delayed compared to cyclophosphamide plus TBI, perhaps diminishing the number pf pancytopenic days post-transplant.

Although potentially of considerable interest, a direct comparison of the conditioning regimens of busulfan plus cyclophosphamide and cyclophosphamide plus TBI has not been reported. In any case, the relapse rate in acute myelogenous leukemia patients transplanted during first remission after conditioning with busulfan plus cyclophosphamide (< 10%) appears to be less than with various cyclophosphamide plus TBI regimens (20–40%). Although busulfan plus cyclophosphamide has not been extensively tested in hematologic neoplasms other than acute myelogenous leukemia, it would seem to be less attractive for treating lymphoid hematologie neoplasms or those hematologie malignacies that frequently involve the central nervous system. Moreover, this regimen would not seem to be very attractive for chronic myelogenous leukemia patients previously treated with high cumulative doses of busulfan given in conventional schedules, because such patients may be predisposed to an increased incidence of lung toxicity (this may be a problem with those patients given TBI as well). Therefore, this regimen appears to be primarily useful in cases of acute myelogenous leukemia.

BACT and Variants

In an attempt to avoid the toxicity of TBI the BACT regimen (BCNU [carmustine] plus arabinosyl cytosine plus cyclophosphamide plus thioguanine) was developed at the National Cancer Institute (U.S.) in the 1970s. Subsequently, this regimen was found to be ineffective for the conditioning of patients with acvanced acute leukemia, but to have some utility in the treatment of certain lymphomas (notably Burkitt's lymphoma), especially with autologous marrow transplants.

At the present time, BACT has been extensively modified and is used only infrequently as designed, save perhaps in Burkitt's lymphoma patients. BACT has been modified to CBV (cyclophosphamide, BCNU and VP16-213 [etoposide]), a regimen used to treat Hodgkin's disease, primarily with autologous marrow transplants. Numerous other modifications have been developed and are undergoing clinical use.

Conditioning for Second Transplants

In general, second transplants are considered in two circumstances: graft rejection for aplastic anemia and (late) systemic recurrence of hematologic malignancy. While both situations are desperate, the latter is usually more so, since conditioning for aplastic anemia is rarely so intensive or cumulatively toxic that a second course of conditioning can not be given. The problem with leukemia is different. First, presumably the most active regimen was used initially, and a second, less effective regimen must therefore be asked to do what the first could not. (However, this is not invariably the case, as some "good-risk" patients transplanted in an initial remission may have received a regimen of less than "maximal" activity and toxicity.) Second, especially since many leukemia patients will have been exposed to tissue-tolerance levels of total body irradiation, cumulative toxicity (especially to the lung) may be present. This feature both precludes safe administration of a second course of total body irradiation, and also possibly increases the risk of pneumonitis even for conditioning regimens without TBI.

In designing a policy for second transplants, it is obvious that only selected patients should be considered. In general, those patients with a stable clinical status who can reasonably be expected to have greater success with a second conditioning regimen are the most attractive. Also, those patients who did not experience severe toxicity from the first transplant are probably the best candidates. This statement especially applies to patients who had severe graft-vs-host disease with the first transplant; they are less desirable candidates, especially if they had non-malignant disease and would not benefit from the "favorable" aspect of graft-vs-host disease, i.e., graft-vs-leukemia.

Given these considerations, most aplastic patients who reject but are in reasonable shape should be regarded as candidates for second transplants with more intensive conditioning. Conditioning may be accomplished using either irradiation, antihymocyte globulin, posttransplant therapy with buffy-coat infusions or cyclosporine, or combinations of the above. Conversely, leukemia patients should be highly selected. The following guidelines may form the basis of such a consideration:

1. Disease-free interval of greater than one year after initial transplant;
2. Initial transplantation in an early remission;
3. The availability of a conditioning regimen that offers both active agents not used previously, and those not likely to produce excessive non-hematologic toxicity. For example, busulfan plus cyclophosphamide could be used after cyclophosphamide plus TBI, or vice versa. (A very aggressive approach would attempt to augment the graft-vs-host and -leukemia reactions, especially in patients who had not experienced them previously.)

In summary, second marrow transplantation is not routine, and is unlikely to become so in the near future, especially for leukemics. In this regard, it should be remembered that some leukemic patients may have successful palliation and, rarely, prolonged survival with convention chemotherapy alone.

Approaches to Improving Results of Conditioning Regimens

Development of New Conditioning Regimens

General considerations. Unless a formal clinical research study is planned, it is prudent to use an established conditioning regimen rather than to construct a novel regimen for use in a few patients. Such efforts are generally not worthwhile, in part because they are usually applied to a high-risk population not suitable for standard conditioning regimens, and because the resultant poor outcome is likely to produce neither benefit to the patient nor useful data to the investigator. If modifications of an existing conditioning regimen are deemed essential in a particular case, minimal deviations from the standard regimen are recommended.

Although many different conditioning regimens have been tested during the past decade, there have been few studies specifically designed to determine the superiority of a given regimen. While it is difficult to perform such randomized trials, the importance of optimal conditioning regimens makes it surprising that more have not been undertaken.

The need to develop new conditioning regimens, especially for the hematologic malignancies, in some respects depends upon one's view of the role of marrow transplantation in these diseases. For example, if marrow transplantation for leukemia is only used to consolidate the first remission state, it will be very difficult to justify a more intensive conditioning regimen. Not only would it be difficult to prove a reduction in recurrence without entering several hundred patients into a randomized clinical trial, but any increase in toxicity might offset potential augmentation of antileukemic efforts. On the other hand, if marrow transplant regimens are used mainly in patients who fail primary chemotherapy, then alternative tactics, e.g. intensification of current conditioning regimens, will undoubtedly be important.

In reality, neither approach is universally applicable. For example, marked improvements in curability with primary therapy would suggest marrow transplantation to be most useful as a salvage therapy, unless subgroups with a poor prognosis could be identified while in an initial remission. On the other hand, if they become markedly safer, marrow transplant regimens may continue to be useful as consolidation therapy in an initial remission, since they tend to be more effective than conventional regimens. In any case, development of improved conditioning regimens will likely be important for the foreseeable future.

Specific considerations. In the construction of a new regimen, several factors deserve consideration:

1. The goal in construction a new regimen is to improve survival, and a correlation exists between dose-intensity and toxicity. For instance, a regimen of greater intensity is expected to produce better antitumor effects, but perhaps at the cost of more toxicity. This was the case with the potent antileukemic regimen SCARI (thioguanine, cyclophosphamide, cytarabine, daunorubicin, and TBI), where the decreased relapse rate of acute leukemics who underwent allogeneic marrow transplantation after SCARI was negated by an increased number of toxic deaths. Therefore, mere augmentation of doses of current components may not be very useful. Conversely, this argument should not be interpreted to conclude that more effective regimens that are necessarily more toxic. The point to be emphasized is that a systematic approach to this problem is required, and the development of these improved regimens may prove difficult.

   Similarly, while considerations of toxicity or the use of cycle specific agents suggest conditioning regimens should extend over several days, they should in fact be administered over no more than 7–10 days. Longer intervals will expose patients to the risks of prolonged pancytopenia. This was a specific problem with SCARI, which required 2.5 weeks to administer; the subsequent period of prolonged neutropenia contributed to the high rate of infectious deaths noted with SCARI. On the other hand, the often unpredictable non-hematologic toxicity of the agents used in escalated doses makes the sumultaneous use of these agents less attracitve as compared to their administration on separate days.

2. While it will be difficult to develop unique conditioning regimens for each disease, especially malignancies, it is also difficult to believe that a single regimen will be optimal for all diseases. As a general rule, conditioning used for antineoplastic effects should not contain elements used in the primary therapy, both to avoid cumulative toxicity and especially to minimize the exposure of resistant malignant cell populations to previously-used agents. Considering the agents new used in primary therapy for hematologic malignancies, and the fact that the toxicity (especially myelosuppression) of some agents given at high doses is excessive for conventional use, the most attractive currently-available elements for the construction of improved of new conditioning regimens for hematologic cancer include busulfan, melphalan and TBI. Carmustine (BCNU) is also potentially attractive, but in high doses it produces serious overlapping non-hematologic toxicities with other agents, especially interstitial pneumonitis. High-dose cytosine arabinoside or etoposide may also be useful, especially if they are not part of conventional treatment regimens. Cyclophosphamide is less attractive in that it is often used in conventional therapy regimens, but still fulfills certain of these criteria. Moreover, cyclophosphamide lacks overlapping non-hematologic toxicity with busulfan, TBI, BCNU and melphalan, and its effectiveness in combinations has been well established over almost two decades of use.

   A nagging concern in the development of improved conditioning regimens is the possibility that a truly useful drug has been overlooked in previous drug-development studies. Specifically, current elements are usually drugs used in conventional chemotherapy albeit at augmented doses. It is possible that active but very myelosuppressive agents, unsuitable for conventional chemotherapy but ideal for conditioning regimens for marrow transplantation, have been excluded from further evaluation at a very early phase of development. Likewise, there is always the question of whether an agent that is not very active in conventional doses may be useful in escalated doses for conditioning. While the use of such agents are somewhat attractive, their use is also encompasses a long development period, i.e. formal Phase I-II trial sequence.

   Finally, it is not necessary that all agents in a conditioning regimen be used in augmented doses. The use of some agents in conventional dose might be considered for patients in whom a particularly desirable agent did not lend itself to dose escalation but which was not extensively used in primary therapy. The use of additional agents in this manner may minimize toxicity.

3. If the regimen is to be used for allogeneic marrow transplantation, a potent immunosuppressive element is required. As noted earlier, while this is neither necessary nor desirable for syngeneic or autologous bone marrow transplantation regimens, it may be critical to use a potently immunosuppressive regimen for durable engraftment in certain situations, e.g., T-cell depletion in histoincompatible transplants.

4. In certain circumstances, the superiority of a new versus a standard regimen will be difficult to prove. For instance, determining of relative effectiveness of standard versus test regimens will require a large randomized trial unless one regimen is strikingly more effective. The problem of patient numbers is complicated in the case of allogeneic marrow transplants, in which a high death rate due to non-malignant (and frequently inevaluable) problems can be anticipated. However, with the non-hematologic malignancies in which complete remissions are usually infrequent, these considerations are less applicable. Finally, despite the difficulty in carrying out such studies the importance of randomized trials is re-emphasized; the evolution of primary conventional therapeutic pre-transplantation will produce a non-uniform patient population that may generate erroneous conclusions in non-randomized trials performed sequentially.

Given the high incidence of malignant disease recurrence, efforts to improve the therapeutic index of current conditioning regimens for diseases such as leukemia concentrate primarily on augmenting their antitumor efficacy. However, although survival could be increased by a reduction in toxicity, decreasing the dosage of toxic elements, is probably not an advisable approach in most situations. Specifically, recurrence is usually the chief cause of death, and since at least a rough correlation exists between intensity, antileukemic efficacy and toxicity, increased recurrences might result. Nevertheless, such a relationship should not be accepted as inevitable, and a reduction in the toxicity of the conditioning regimen would be especially welcome if no concomitant increase in recurrence rates were observed.

A salient question regarding both efficacy and safety concerns the need for TBI. For instance, there are definite limitations on TBI dose as TBI clearly contributes to severe and often fatal (especially pulmonary) toxicity. In certain diseases, these problems are amplified. For instance, the malignant lymphomas (both Hodgkin's disease and the intermediate- and high-grade non-Hodgkin's lymphomas) are being transplanted more frequently. Based on conventinal fractionation schedules, many lymphomas require relatively high doses to prevent recurrence, suggesting the much lower cumulative doses achievable with single-fraction TBI are not likely to be very effective. Also, many conventional anti-lymphoma regimens, especially those for Hodgkin's disease, include previous therapy with mediastinal radiotherapy (and perhaps bleomycin) that produce subclinical lung damage, predisposing patients to an increased risk of interstitial pneumonia after transplantation.

For these reasons, a large number of regimens that do not use TBI have been developed. As expected, intensive single-agent chemotherapy has not been very successful, although high-dose melphalan ($\geq$ 140 mg/m^2) requiring marrow support has produced some durable remissions in both hematologic and non-hematologic tumors. However, these non-TBI regimens have had only variable success; the busulfan plus cyclophosphamide regimen for acute myelogenous leukemia, and to a lesser extent certain of the various modifications of BACT (such as CBV), are perhaps the chief exceptions to this statement. Given the variety of agents with antineoplastic activity in general clinical use, it seems reasonable to evaluate combination chemotherapy regimens that do not include TBI. This is expecially the case for the various solid malignancies that are relatively insensitive to radiation.

A number of combinations of the agents listed in Table 9 have been experimented with. By and large, however, these combinations have not been tested in a manner that permits a critical evaluation of their relative efficacy. (This statement applies not only to relatively minor modifications but even to major additions or deletions.) Nevertheless, one is left with the impression that these regimens have roughly the same level of efficacy, although they manifest differences in toxicity. Since these regimens use mainly the same agents, it may be assumed that innovative regimens will be required to improve results, particularly in patients with most advances hematologic malignancies and probably all non-hematologic cancers.

However, it should not be assumed that TBI is intrinsically undesirable. TBI has many positive attributes, chief among them its ability to kill drug-resistant cells. Given its substantial toxicity when used in doses close to maximal, an alternative strategy is suggested. Instead of using TBI in high dose to kill the majority of cells, perhaps it should be used only to obliterate those cells truly resistant to chemotherapy. This strategy might permit a lower, less toxic dose of TBI to be used.

Post-transplantation Therapy

In some respects, therapy given after transplantation is attractive, as a minimal tumor burden exists in patients at high risk to ultimately experience a recurrence of disease. For several reasons, however, conventional modalities employed post-transplant are not very attractive. Most importantly, the status of the transplanted marrow (and the patient as well) is fragile in the early post-grafting period; this precludes myelosuppressive therapy, which would probably produce unacceptable toxicity. Were such treatment delayed until a stable clinical and marrow status was attained, it would undoubtedly be less toxic, but it would also be less effective in terms of preventing recurrence of residual tumor. A possible exception to this statement is a treatment involving more than one course of conditioning and transplantation. While attractive in theory, the limitation with this tactic is cumulative toxicity, usually non-hematologic, but also hematologic if marrow is collected between courses (see III.3). In general, conditioning remains a "one shot" proposition.

However, less myelosuppressive therapies are more attractive. For instance, manipulation of the "graft-vs-leukemia" effect (detailed in IV and V) as a post-transplant modality has some positive features. Unfortunately, in man this effect also seems to parallel graft-vs-host disease, a process of major morbidity and mortality, and it is likely that few workers in allogeneic bone marrow transplantation would miss the graft-vs-leukemia effect were graft-vs-host disease eliminated! However, morbidity and mortality are more endemic to acute than chronic graft-vs-host disease; perhaps the latter could be provoked in a mild form that would be actively antileukemic without being excessively toxic. In any case, the ability to precisely modulate either of these processes is currently very limited.

In this context, various modifiers of biologic responses may be considered. Potential agents include the interferons, tumor necrosis factor, monoclonal antibodies conjugated with drugs, radiopharmaceuticals and other toxins. These agents could, of course, be used before transplantation, but since they often are administered over a relatively long period and have variable but often minimal myelosuppression, their use after transplantation is also feasible.

Pre-conditioning Cytoreduction

It is important to consider the role of conventional therapy used to produce initial cytoreduction before transplantation. (For a variety of reasons, transplantation has only rarely been employed as primary therapy, usually in circumstances in which the usual primary therapy is ineffective in producing initial remissions.) Primary conventional therapy usually is often not detailed or considered in reports on the efficacy of transplantation, but may be of critical importance; while the degree of cytoreduction achieved with conventional chemotherapy is rarely known, the residual tumor burden or "depth" of remission is presumably a major factor in determining the subsequent success of conditioning regimens. Patients in a "shallow" remission (or relapse) may simply have too much tumor for it to be eradicated by even a potent conditioning regimen. Also, there is evidence in the acute leukemias that conventional chemotherapy and conditioning regimens used with transplantation are at least partially non-cross-resistant, suggesting that optimal use of the former contributes to the apparent success of the latter.

Moreover, it is not widely appreciated that changes in conventional primary therapy potentially produce profoundly different situations in patients for therapy with conditioning regimens for marrow transplantation. In addition to the consideration in the above paragraph, it is reasonable to assume that conventional therapies are usually less toxic than intensive conditioning (even when the latter are accompanied by marrow support), and that the former will always be preferred if effective. In this case, conventional therapies improve, the use of transplantation to consolidate initial remissions will become less attractive. Moreover, the failures of such improved conventional primary regimens will be more resistant to existing conditioning regimens, and will therefore be associated with poorer results.

In any event, observations to date do not clearly support the use of additional conventional chemotherapy to consolidate remissions before transplantation, or even to produce remission from the relapsed state. Although it is difficult to generalize, in a previously-treated patient the tumor status at the time of referral to the transplant center should usually be accepted and patients transplanted promptly. The use of additional conventional chemotherapy may or may not significantly enhance cell kill, but is likely to produce cumulative toxicity predisposing the patient to complications that may compromise or obviate transplantation.

However, there are exceptions to the recommendation to accept the tumor status at the time of referral. For example, modalities other than conventional systemic chemotherapy are available to reduce tumor load. Bulk tumor deposits (especially lymphomatous) in the central nervous system, gonads or lymph nodes may be treated with local radiotherapy that does not enhance systemic therapy. (However, conventional involved-field radiotherapy to the mediastinum should be avoided if a conditioning regimen including TBI is planned, as several studies have indicated that such therapy predisposes to fatal interstitial pneumonitis.) Intrathecal chemotherapy to control meningeal leukemia may be considered in much the same manner. While these tactics are unlikely to be evaluated definitively by randomized clinical trials, their use is especially reasonable when local relapse rates are excessive with standard conditioning regimens alone. Nevertheless, as a pragmatic approach, one should probably administer conventional primary therapy to those patients with disease that can be reliably induced into remission and immediately transplant those who do not have such treatment available.

Finally, it follows that the effects of both conventional chemotherapy and marrow transplantation regimens will be difficult to assess as long as patients do not have standardized therapy. For example, while even leukemic patients may have very different tumor loads in first remission even if they have received identical induction therapy varying primary therapies will amplify these differences. Consideration should be given to the use of a standard remission induction therapy (as well as intensive conditioning) and, ultimately, to randomized trials of these components. Moreover, if it is very likely that a transplant will be performed as initial consolidation, primary therapy may eventually be tailored to permit the most definitive conditioning therapy to be administered.

Future of Conditioning Regimens

Although it would be easy to conclude that in the future "new" agents, either previously unused existing cytotoxic drugs or perhaps truly unique agents, might be available to produce improvement conditioning regimens, this will not necessarily be the case. For instance, while it is clear that current modifications of the cyclophosphamide and single-fraction TBI regimen are more convenient to administer and perhaps slightly more effective, it would be difficult to conclude that the classic cyclophosphamide and unfractionated TBI regimen used by Dr. Thomas' group in 1970 is grossly inappropriate as therapy for selected patients. (Whether this is due to the intrinsic excellence of this regimen or the lack of a firm direction in the sequential evaluation of conditioning regimens is speculative.) Of course, one obviously hopes for new components to improve the therapeutic index of conditioning; however, it is to be emphasized that the most immediate way to improve survival for the largest number of transplanted patients would be to decrease leukemic recurrence rates. In the absence of strikingly improved new regimens, this goal could be attained in part by providing optimal, standardized initial therapy to all suitable patients and by performing marrow transplantation at the earliest appropriate moment.

References

Appelbaum FR, Clift RA, Buckner CD, et al. (1983) Allogeneic marrow transplantation for acute nonlymphoblastic leukemia after first relapse. Blood 61: 949

Appelbaum FR, Dahlberg S, Thomas ED, et al. (1984) Bone marrow transplantation or chemotherapy after remission induction for adults with acute nonlymphoblastic leukemia. Ann Int Med 101: 581

Appelbaum FR, Storb R, Ranberg RE, et al. (1984) Allogeneic marrow transplantation in the treatment of preleukemia. Ann Int Med 100: 689

Atkinson K, Biggs J, Concannon A, et al. (1986) Second marrow transplant for recurrence of haematological malignancy. Bone Marrow Transplant 1: 159

Badger C, Buckner CD, Thomas ED, et al. (1982) Allogeneic marrow transplantation for acute leukemia in relapse. Leuk Res 6: 383

Blume KG, Forman SJ, O'Donnell MR, et al. (1987) Total body irradiation and high-dose etoposide: A new preparatory regimen for bone marrow transplantation in patients with advanced hematologic malignancies. Blood 69: 1015

Fefer A, Cheever MA, Thomas ED, et al. (1981) Bone marrow transplantation for refractory acute leukemia in 34 patients with identical twins. Blood 57: 421

Fischer A, Blanche S, Verber F, et al. (1986) Prevention of graft failure by an anti-HLFA-1 monoclonal antibody in HLA-mismatched bone marrow transplantation. Lancet 2: 1058

Forman SJ, Nademanee AP, O'Donnell MR, et al. (1985) High-dose cytosine arabinoside and daunomycin as primary therapy for adults with acute non-lymphoblastic leukemia: A pilot study. Semin in Oncol 12 (Suppl 2): 114

Gale RP (1984) How does bone marrow transplantation cure leukemia? Lancet 2: 28

Gale RP (1985) Progress in acute myelogenous leukemia. Ann Int Med 101: 702

Herzig RH, Coccia PF, Lazarus HM, et al. (1985) Bone marrow transplantation for acute leukemia and lymphoma with high-dose cytosine arabinoside and total body irradiation. Semin in Oncol 12 (Suppl 3): 184

Jagannath S, Dicke KA, Armitage JO, et al. (1986) High-dose cyclophosphamide, carmustine, and etoposide and autologous bone marrow transplantation for relapsed Hodgkin's disease. Ann Int Med 104: 163

Messner HA, Curtis JE, Minden MM (1985) The combined use of cytosine arabinoside, cyclophosphamide and total body irradiation as a preparative regimen for bone marrow transplantation in patients with acute chronic and myelogenous leukemia. Semin in Oncol 12 (Suppl 3): 187

Parkman R, Rappeport JM, Hellman S, et al. (1984) Busulfan and total body irradiation as antihematopoietic stem cell agents in the preparation of patients with congenital bone marrow disorders for allogeneic bone marrow transplantation. Blood 64: 852

Ramsay NKC, Kim TH, McGlave P, et al. (1983) Total lymphoid irradiation and cyclophosphamide conditioning prior to bone marrow transplantation. Blood 62: 622

Santos GW (1987) Preparative regimens for allogeneic bone marrow transplantation in leukemia. In Gale RP and Champlin R (eds.). Progress in Bone Marrow Transplantation. NY, Alan R. Liss, Inc., pp 113

Santos GW, Tutschka P, Brookmeyer R, et al. (1983) Marrow transplantation for acute nonlymphocytic leukemia after treatment with busulfan and cyclophosphamide. N Engl J Med 309: 1347

Slavin S (1987) Total lymphoid irradiation. Immunology 8: 88

Storb R, Doney KC, Thomas ED, et al. (1982) Marrow transplantation with or without donor buffy coat cells for 65 transfused aplastic anemia patients. Blood 59: 236

Storb R, Thomas ED, Buckner CD, et al. (1980) Marrow transplantation in thirty "untransfused" patients with severe aplastic anemia. Ann Intern Med 92: 30

Thomas ED (1982) The use and potential of bone marrow allograft and whole-body irradiation in the treatment of leukemias. Cancer 50: 1449

Thomas ED (1986) The role of marrow transplantation in malignant disease. Cancer 49: 1963

Thomas ED, Clift RA, Hosman G, et al. (1982) Marrow transplantation for acute nonlymphoblastic leukemia in first remission using fractionated or single-dose irradiation. Int J Rad Oncol Biol Phys 8: 817

VanBekkum DW (1984) Conditioning regimens for marrow grafting. Semin Hematol 21(2): 81

3. Collection, Processing and Infusion of Marrow

The preparative or conditioning regimen (see above, III. 2) before marrow infusion creates space for the transfused donor marrow. Through mechanisms not yet completely understood, intravenously infused donor marrow cells reseed in the bone marrow cavity ("homing") of the recipient and start to replicate and differentiate. The cell type that is acutally transplanted is the pluripotent progenitor cell ("stem cell") capable of self renewal and differentiation.

How is the Marrow Obtained?

Bone marrow harvesting is performed under sterile conditions in the operating room, usually by two members of the transplant team. The whole procedure requires about 1–2 hours with the donor under general anesthesia. In patients with contraindications for general anesthesia, epidural anesthesia can be performed instead. Sites of bone marrow aspiration are mainly the posterior and anterior iliac crests. The practice of using just the posterior pelvis has the advantage of shortening the procedure time by the need to turn the donor. Sometimes marrow is also taken from the sternum, particularly where a large marrow dose is desired, as in patients with aplastic anemia or when there is a major size disparity between donor (small) and recipient (large). In children who serve as donors for adult patients, the upper third of the tibiae may also be used for aspiration. On the average, $2–10 \times 10^8$ mononuclear cells/kg are harvested for an allogeneic marrow graft, and about $1–3 \times 10^8$ cells/kg for an autologous marrow graft. Increasing donor age is associated with a reduction in the number of nucleated cells collected, and therefore a larger volume may be required from older donors.

The risks for the donor are largely confined to those of anesthesia. An analysis of over 1200 marrow donors revealed only 6 serious incidents, predominantly related to general anesthesia. Spinal anesthesia can cause postspinal headache and occasionally urinary retention. Prolonged bleeding from the marrow harvest site or infections occur rarely, and the hospitalization time for the donor is, on an average, one to two days. Usually the donor does not require any blood support perioperatively. Some centers, however, prefer to store autologous blood, which can be transfused during marrow harvest. This prevents the donor from being at risk for transfusion acquired diseases in case transfusions during or after the procedure are required. In the above quoted study from Seattle the proportion of donors who, in addition to the infusion of stored autologous blood during the harvest, required allogeneic red cell transfusion after the marrow harvest was 1% of males and 8% of females. No data are available on patients who do not receive autologous red cell transfusion.

The needles used for marrow harvesting are 6–10 cm long with a ball or knob handle (Fig. 2). Prior to the procedure, the aspiration syringes are rinsed with a solution consisting of medium mixed with heparin. Through puncture sites in the skin, about 5–10 aspirations are performed with the needle point being moved a few millimeters for each aspiration. While the needle is rotated to expose the bevel to different areas of bone marrow, vigorous suction is applied. In order to get the required number of nucleated cells, about 150–250 aspirations need to be done. It is advisable not to take more than 2–4 ml from a single location since the amount of peripheral blood may otherwise increase, thereby reducing the relative number of nucleated marrow cells, and increasing the number of peripheral blood cells. The marrow is then expelled into a beaker (Fig. 2) containing heparinized tissue culture medium.

After marrow aspiration is completed the marrow is passed through coarse and fine mesh filters into a second beaker (Fig. 2). This filtration step is required to remove bone fragments and fat particles from the marrow that might cause

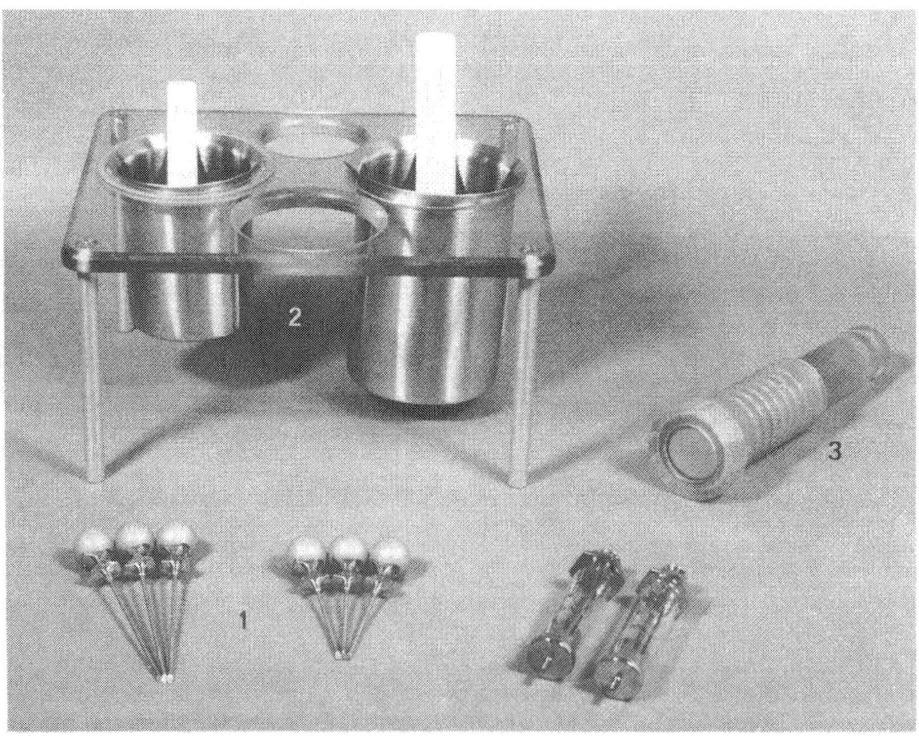

Fig. 2. Marrow aspiration equipment including needles and glass syringes (1), stand with beakers (2) and screen (3)

pulmonary emboli in the recipient. When marrow samples have been taken for culture and cell counting, the marrow is placed into a standard blood transfer pack for infusion into the patient.

Marrow Infusion

The harvested marrow may remain untreated or may be transferred to the laboratory for T-cell depletion or other forms of marrow purging (see below). If the harvested marrow is not processed further it will be immediately transferred from the operating room to the transplantation ward and prepared for infusion. However, if no immediate transfusion is possible, for instance when donor and patient are located in different cities, the marrow can be kept viable in the cold for some time. Although no exact data exist as to how long human marrow can be kept fresh, successful engraftment has been obtained with marrow stored at 4° C for up to 48 hours after harvesting. All nonessential medication and transfusions on the day of marrow infusion should be avoided to prevent interference with the infused marrow or to cover-up side effects of marrow infusion.

A large bore central venous catheter (usually a Hickman line), is preferred for marrow infusion which usually requires about 2–4 hours. Side effects during marrow infusion are not common. In an occasional patient, transient mild cyanosis with tachycardia can occur due to multiple small lung emboli caused by tiny clumps of bone marrow cells. Mild hemolysis secondary to ABO-incompatibilities is sometimes observed, especially when isoagglutinins of the patient are not completely removed by plasma exchange before transplantation (see III.2). In very small recipients, marrow infusion may result in volume overload, which can usually be controlled by the administration of diuretics or may require apheresis of a corresponding volume of peripheral blood.

Marrow Storage

Malignant lymphomas and solid tumors may not involve the bone marrow, and this "clean" marrow can then be harvested and stored for later use. In patients with acute leukemia, marrow for autologous transplantation can be taken in first remission and stored for later reinfusion, either in a subsequent relapse or remission. For marrow storage, nucleated-cell buffy coat is removed from the marrow by centrifugation in a standard blood-transfer pack using devices such as the IBM 2991 or Sorvall RC-3B centrifuges. The buffy coat is resuspended in medium mixed with 10% dimethyl-sulfoxide as a cryoprotective agent, and placed in plastic bags made of polyolefine. These bags are frozen in a controlled rate freezer at $-1°$ C per minute to a temperature of $-60°$ C and at $-5°$ C per minute to a temperature of $-90°$ C and then transferred to the liquid phase of a liquid-nitrogen freezer. On the day of autologous marrow transfusion the bags are thawed rapidly in a water bath at 37° C and transfused immediately with a rate of about 15–20 ml per minute. Some loss in viability and cell number can occur with the freezing and thawing procedure. Therefore, cell viability before and after freezing has to be determined. Recovery of hematopoietic stem cell function after freezing and thawing should be on the order of 90% of fresh cells. In addition, cultures should be taken before freezing and after thawing, to exclude bacterial and fungal contamination of the stored marrow.

At some centers *double* (tandem) autologous marrow transplantation is performed: marrow is reharvested during the early regeneration phase following the first autograft, when tumor contamination is expected to be minimal, and the transplant procedure is then repeated. Frozen marrow can be used for successful marrow transplants after many years of storage. In a recent study, marrow recovery was possible with autologous marrow stored more than five years.

Manipulation (Purging) of (Donor) Marrow

Several modalities for in vitro treatment ("purging") of the harvested marrow have been developed in order to remove either T-cells from the donor marrow (T-cell depletion), or malignant cells from the patient's own marrow (tumor cell purging). For these procedures the marrow is taken to the laboratory where the manipulation is to be performed. Red blood cells and mononuclear cells can be separated either by conventional Ficoll-Hypaque technique of by the use of special centrifuges or cell washers (e.g. IBM 2991).

T-cell depletion: (Table 11; see also IV.2.) Most commonly T-cells from the donor marrow are removed by monoclonal antibodies against T-cells with or without the use of complement (cytolytic treatment). Instead of complement, immunotoxins such as ricin chain A conjugated to monoclonal antibodies are now being employed. Donor T-cells can also be removed by lectin agglutination or by the use of magnetic beads coated with monoclonal antibodies against T-cell surface antigens. In addition, some mechanical methods such as density gradient centrifugation, and counterflow elutriation are being developed (see IV.2).

Tumor cell purging: When the patient's own (autologous) marrow is used for transplantation, there is always concern that clonogenic leukemia, lymphoma or

Table 11. Methods of In Vitro T-Cell Depletion

Opsonization with
– Heterologous antisera
– Monoclonal antibodies
Density gradients
Monoclonal antibodies and complement
Monoclonal antibodies coupled to
– Magnetic beads
– Immunotoxins
Lectin (soybean) agglutination
Counterflow elutriation
Chemoseparation

other malignant cells are present and upon reinfusion could lead to recurrent disease. Consequently attempts are being made to remove residual tumor cells by immunological, pharmacological or physical techniques ("purging"). This can be achieved with monoclonal antibodies directed at malignant B-cell or T-cell markers. Alternatively in vitro cytotoxic drugs may be used, such as 4-hydroxy-perpoxy-cyclophosphamide (Mafosfamide), a derivative of cyclophosphamide aimed at destroying malignant cells.

For purging purposes a buffy coat of nucleated cells is separated from the marrow. This cell fraction is then mixed with autologous plasma and a culture medium/heparin mixture along with the corresponding monoclonal antibody or cytotoxic drug at 37° C for 30 minutes. In case of monoclonal antibody treatment, a second incubation with complement is needed to lyse the target cells, followed by several washing steps, before the marrow can be frozen or reinfused into the recipient. Purging procedures have to be done on fresh marrow, thawed marrow is not suitable for this procedure.

Long term culture: For patients with CML or AML, long-term in vitro culture may prove to be a useful method. For this purpose, bone marrow is set up for culture using standard culture techniques. After several days in culture, leukemic cells begin to die off – a condition that selects in favor of normal elements. Usually after a period of 10 days, this leukemia cell-free autologous marrow can either be reinfused into the patient or stored frozen for later use. Although still experimental, this technique offers exciting therapeutic avenues specifically for patients who do not have an HLA identical donor.

Back-up Marrow

The term "back-up marrow" refers to a fraction of the aspirated marrow which, in the case of marrow manipulation, remains untreated. If the purged autologous marrow is contaminated, or engraftment is not achieved, the back-up fraction can be used to salvage the patient. The bulk, i.e. about 75% of the collected marrow, is usually used for purging procedures. The remainder ($\geq 1 \times 10^8$ nucleated cells/kg) is cryopreserved and held in reserve.

Cryopreservation of an autologous back-up marrow may also be useful if mismatched T-cell depleted related or unrelated marrow transplantation is performed since these transplants carry an increased risk of graft rejection.

Peripheral Blood Stem Cell Transplantation

From several animal models it is known that hematopoietic progenitor cells, capable of repopulating an aplastic marrow, circulate in peripheral blood. These stem cells can be recovered from peripheral blood by leukapheresis. Using a continous-flow cell separator usually 6–10 sessions are necessary. The leukapheresed nucleated cells, which also contain the stem cell fraction, can be frozen and stored as described above. Peripheral stem cells are usually collected for autologous transplants. The best time to perform an autologous stem cell harvest is usually at the time of "rebound" after chemotherapy, although some centers try to harvest stem cells without preceding chemotherapy (see IV.3.). The procedure is work intensive because it requires staff for repeated leukapheresis and freezing, but has the advantage of not requiring general anesthesia of the donor. This might be of potential value if donors are at risk for complications due to general anesthesia. Furthermore, some patients, especially those with malignant lymphoma, may have received irradiation of the pelvis during induction or consolidation treatment, and the yield from pelvic bone is not sufficient. For these patients, stem cell transplantation may offer a therapeutic option. Although not proven, it could become possible to use peripheral stem cell transplantation for patients who have marrow involvement of the underlying disease without signs of any active disease in the peripheral blood such as patients with multiple myeloma. Although still speculative, this procedure might then be used instead of autologous marrow grafting and purging of the marrow before reinfusion. This form of transplantation may also become an option for the allogeneic setting.

Transplantation of Cadaveric Marrow

A cadaveric source of bone marrow is attractive in view of the fact that many patients do not have a suitable living donor. The availability of cadaveric marrow, which must be taken shortly after death and subsequently frozen and stored, might circumvent this shortage. So far, only one case of successful engraftment with cadaveric marrow (father → son) has been reported, and many hurdles will have to be overcome. However, the procedure seems to be possible; it awaits further testing and refining.

Technically, the outer cortex of both iliac bones is removed with an electrical bone saw, and the trabecular bone marrow containing red marrow can then be extracted using a bone press. Marrow may also be obtained from the lumbar spine. Samples are cut into small pieces, and stirred with medium for about 30 minutes to release bone marrow cells. After passing through a stainless steel sieve, the cells are layered over Ficoll-Hypaque and processed further for T-cell depletion and storage.

Allogeneic marrow transplantation is still a very complex issue, dependent upon a suitable donor. To make this treatment option available to more patients, some of the described developments need to become more routinely available in the future, thus fascilitating bone marrow transplantation. The overall goal, of course, would be to have a universal donor, i. e. a source of marrow available to everyone who would benefit from this procedure.

References

Bell AJ, Hamblin TJ, Oscier DG (1987) Peripheral blood stem cell autografting. Haematol Oncol 5: 45

Blazar BR, Lasky LC, Perentesis JP, Watson KV, Steinberg SE, Filipovich AH, Orr HT, Ramsay NKC (1986) Successful donor cell engraftment in a recipient of bone marrow from a cadaveric donor. Blood 67: 1655

Buckner CD, Clift RA, Sanders JE, Stewart P, Bensinger WI, Doney KC, Sullivan KM, Witherspoon RP, Deeg HJ, Appelbaum FR, Storb R, Thomas ED (1984) Marrow harvesting from normal donors. Blood 64: 630

Coulombel L, Kalousek DK, Eaves CJ, Gupta CM, Eaves AC (1983) Long-term marrow culture reveals chromosomally normal hematopoietic progenitor cells in patients with Philadelphia chromosome-positive chronic myelogneous leukemia. N Eng J Med 308: 1493

Gorin NC (1986) Collection, manipulation and freezing of haemopoietic stem cells. Clinics in Haematol 15(1): 19

Körbling M, Dorken B, Ho AD, Pezutto A, Hunstein W, Fliedner TM (1986) Autologous transplantation of blood derived hemapoietic stem cells after myeloablative therapy in a patient with Burkitt's lymphoma. Blood 67: 529

Thomas ED, Storb R (1970) Technique for human marrow grafting. Blood 36: 507

Treleaven JG, Kemshead JT (1985) Removal of tumor cells from bone marrow: an evaluation of the available techniques. Haematol Oncol 3: 65

IV. Acute Transplant Related Problems

1. Side Effects of Conditioning

Overview

Despite the reconstitutive effects of marrow transplantation, severe (and occasionally even irreversible) toxicity inevitably occurs. The severe hematologic toxicity produced by conditioning is usually manifest by the day of transplantation (day 0). The resultant pancytopenia, although eventually reversible in the vast majority of cases, predisposes to neutropenic infection and thrombocytopenic hemorrhage at least until count recovery ensues (2–3 weeks after the transplant). Somewhat longer is required for counts to reach normal levels. However, there are special circumstances in which rejection or poor graft function cause prolonged cytopenia, i.e., some cases of aplastic anemia, histoincompatible transplants (especially when T-cell depletion has been used) and some autologous transplants (especially those in heavily pretreated patients or those with acute myelogenous leukemia). Infectious complications and their management is discussed in Section IV.3.

Some non-hematologic toxicities are frequently seen soon after conditioning is given, while others may be manifested only years later. The early non-hematologic toxicities are discussed in this section.

While most of the early toxicity noted after transplantation is related to the conditioning regimen, it is difficult to differentiate the effects of this from those produced by complications of other processes related to marrow transplantation, i.e., graft-vs-host disease (GVHD), various infections, and the therapies designed to prevent or treat these problems (e.g., cyclosporine, intravenous hyperalimentation and various antibiotics). A pragmatic method to dissect the contribution of conditioning for certain of these complications can be approximated by comparing the effects of different conditioning regimens in patients receiving a constant marrow source and supportive care. For example, the effects of total body irradiation (TBI) regimens may be assessed by evaluating patients who receive allogeneic marrow transplants following conditioning with cyclophosphamide alone or cyclophosphamide plus TBI. However, such comparisons may ignore the variable of diagnosis, as TBI-containing regimens are often used to condition patients with malignant disease, whereas an attempt is made to avoid TBI as conditioning for non-malignant disease. While intrinsic features of a disease may or may not contribute to the early toxicity noted after conditioning, prior exposure to cytotoxic agents used in conventional therapy (e.g., anthracyclines, busulfan, cis-platin), may produce cumulative subclinical damage that becomes apparent only after conditioning and the transplant. In any event, it is probable that most of the complications discussed below as due to conditioning are multifactorial. An example is that of cytomegalovirus interstitial pneumonia; this has been shown to be related to diagnosis, previous therapy (transfusions), conditioning (TBI) and the presence of GVHD.

In any case, there is extensive data on the toxicity of most components of conditioning regimens when used in conventional doses, and more severe toxicity in the same organ system may be assumed with high-dose therapy. In addition, unique toxicities may be seen with high-dose therapy; the cardiotoxicity of cyclophosphamide is an example. This consideration may well apply to augmented-dose combination-therapy conditioning and is a strong reason not to use unique conditioning regimens outside of a clinical research setting.

Specific Complications

These are detailed in Table 12.

Pancytopenia. The most severe complications of pancytopenia, primarily infection and hemorrhage, are considered in detail in Section IV.4.

Table 12. Acute Complications of Marrow Transplantation

- Pancytopenia
- Mucositis and other oral complications
- Gastroenteritis and diarrhea
- Urotoxicity
- Hepatic damage
- Cutaneous toxicity
- Neurotoxicity
- Cardiotoxicity
- Interstitial pneumonitis
- Fluid and electrolyte imbalance

Mucositis and other oral complications. Most conditioning regimens produce some mucositis, usually during the first two weeks after transplantation. The use of high doses of TBI, etoposide, melphalan or thio-tepa will produce more severe mucositis than the use of lower doses of these drugs or other agents. Also, the use of methotrexate as acute GVHD prophylaxis post-transplant will produce or aggravate mucositis.

While mucositis and other oral complications (such as various infections) are not preventable using most current conditioning regimens, these complications may be minimized by correcting pre-existing problems such as partially erupted wisdom teeth and caries. A regular oral hygiene regimen during conditioning and especially the first few weeks after transplantation is likely important. Since secondary infections, especially herpes simplex virus and mucosal candidiasis, are common in this setting, prophylactic systemic acyclovir and topical or especially systemic antifungal agents such as mycostatin and chlortrimazole may be indicated.

When mucositis is first noted, oral feedings and medications should be minimized or discontinued. Cultures should be performed, and treatment begun if a specific infectious agent is identified. Supportive therapy consists of parenteral nutrition and analgesia. While topical anesthesia is helpful in mild cases, opiates often are required for those more severe.

In general, routine consultation with a dentist or oral surgeon is appropriate before initiating the transplant sequence.

Gastroenteritis and diarrhea. In general, agents in the conditioning regimen that produce stomatitis will produce mucosal damage throughout the gastrointestinal tract, the usual manifestation of which is diarrhea. However, diarrhea is a complication that is especially likely to be multifactorial, as a variety of bacterial and viral infections, acute graft-vs-host disease and certain medications may produce a similar clinical picture.

When conditioning has been given, there is little that can be done to prevent subsequent diarrhea. Once diarrhea develops, infectious causes and graft-vs-host disease should be excluded with appropriate cultures and with endoscopy and biopsy if necessary. Oral intake should be minimized or discontinued, and total parenteral nutrition (TPN) is required. Opiates may be helpful for symptomatic control. In addition, the presence of severe diarrhea is an indication that oral drug absorption is unreliable and intravenous medications should be substituted; this statement applies especially to cyclosporine.

Urotoxicity. Hemorrhagic cystitis that occurs after marrow grafting is usually due to acrolein, a toxic metabolite of the drug cyclophosphamide, a common agent of most conditioning regimens. Hemorrhagic cystitis usually appears within two weeks after cyclophosphamide administration. Although hemorrhagic cystitis also occurs later, it is uncertain how frequently this is related to secondary causes such as viral infections, or perhaps graft-versus-host disease. (See IV.7.).

Satisfactory prophylaxis usually can be achieved with hyperhydration, or by using the thiol compound mesna, a uroprotective that binds to acrolein. These measures are outlined in detail in Section IV.7. Neither of the above methods of prophylaxis is completely effective, however. Relatively mild cases of hemorrhagic cystitis can be managed with hyperhydration. Therapeutic platelet transfusion, maintaining levels of 30–50.0 $\times$ 10^9/L may also be useful. Urethral catheterization is indicated if the patient is passing large clots, and in extreme cases, formalin instillation (or even cystectomy) may be required. Obviously, urologic consultation is useful for these more severe cases.

Hepatic damage. Some degree of hepatic damage due to conditioning must be quite common. However, this problem is also very difficult to differentiate from involvement with the underlying disease, systemic infection, hepatitis or damage due to other medications. The most important lesion noted clinically is veno-occlusive disease (VOD) of the liver as discussed in detail in Section IV.6. The complication seems to be more frequent and severe in older patients, and especially in those with pre-existing hepatitis. The usual clinical manifestations of VOD are fluid retention, tender hepatomegaly and jaundice. Although there is no known effective prophylaxis or therapy for VOD, symptomatic control of fluid retention and alertness for signs of liver failure are indicated.

Some conditioning regimens are associated with other hepatic lesions. High doses of carmustine, for example, or occasionally even cyclophosphamide and TBI, can be associated with hepatic necrosis.

Cutaneous toxicity and alopecia. While cyclophosphamide often produces a transient skin rash, severe cutaneous toxicity is rarely due to the conditioning regimen. However, toxic erythema can be seen following the use of high-dose cytarabine or thio-tepa in conditioning regimens. Hyperpigmentation and radiation recall dermatitis can be observed after using many agents.

The proper prophylaxis or therapy for these problems is unknown; however, topical and even systemic steroids may be useful in some cases of high-dose cytarabine toxicity.

Capital alopecia tends to be total, while loss of body hair is more variably. This complication is usually wholly, if slowly reversible.

Neurotoxicity. Leukoencephalopathy is a most serious complication that develops post-transplant, but is usually a chronic rather than an acute disorder (see Section IV.8). Acute complications are usually due to high-dose chemotherapy elements such as the cerebellar toxicity with high-dose cytarabine and the peripheral neuropathy occasionally seen with high-dose etoposide. The former can be prevented somewhat by limiting the use of high-dose cytarabine regimens to younger patients and by using single and cumulative doses less than 3 gm/m^2 and 36 gm/m^2, respectively.

Cardiotoxicity. This complication is mainly noted in patients receiving cyclophosphamide in doses at or above 200 mg/kg. While it is unclear if it is more common in patients whith pre-existing heart disease (due to organic or therapy-related causes), alternatives to the use of cyclophosphamide must be considered in this circumstance. If cyclophosphamide is used, it should never exceed 200 mg/kg.

Interstitial pneumonitis. This term does not relate to a specific disease but rather a clinical, radiographic and histologically-defined syndrome. The best characterized of these processes are infectious in origin, specifically those cases due to cytomegalovirus. However, conditioning (especially that involving TBI), is felt to influence the process denoted as "idiopathic" interstitial pneumonitis, a process in which no other etiology can be defined (see IV.5). There is no specific treatment for this latter process.

Fluid and electrolyte imbalance. Given the copious quantities of intravenous medications (including TPN), required for virtually all transplant patients, the fluid shifts associated with VOD, the nephrotoxicity of antibiotics and cyclosporine, the complex metabolic problems of corticosteroids, and the secondary diarrhea associated with GVHD, it is not surprising that problems of fluid and electrolytes arise soon after marrow transplantation. However, these problems are those generic to very ill patients, and are rarely difficult to correct providing that close monitoring and prompt intervention are routine. Occasionally, dialysis is required, almost exclusively for patients receiving cyclosporine.

Future Directions

Conditioning regimens produce considerable morbidity, and at least contribute to the high mortality rate observed early after transplantation. While a reduction in this toxicity is highly desirable, this goal may not be simple to achieve without a loss of efficacy of conditioning. Specifically, the rough correlation that exists between efficacy and toxicity of conditioning regimens suggests that the most direct method of reducing toxicity i.e., simple dose reduction, is unlikely to improve cure rates.

The most obvious approach to toxicity reduction is less direct. By early transplantation, extensive cumulative toxicity from previous therapy is minimized, and it is likely that some degree of post-transplant toxicity could be avoided.

References

Appelbaum FR, Strauchen JA, Graw RG, et al (1976) Acute lethal carditis caused by high dose combination chemotherapy. Lancet 1: 58

Blacklock H, Ball L, Knight C, et al (1983) Experience with Mesna in patients receiving allogeneic bone marrow transplants for poor prognostic leukemia. Cancer Treat Rev 10 (Suppl A): 45

Brock N. Pohl J. Stekar J (1981) Studies on the urotoxicity of oxazophosphorine cytostatics and its prevention. Eur J Cancer 17: 595

Chaplin RE, Gale RP (1984) The early complications of bone marrow transplantation. Semin Hematol pp 101

Cos PJ (1978) Cyclophosphamide cystitis: Identification of acrolein as the causative agent. Biochem Pharmacol 28: 2045

Freedman A, Ehrlich RM, June BM (1984) Prevention of cyclophosphamide cystitis with 2-mercaptoethane sulfonate: A histologic study. J Uro 132: 580

Gottdiener JS, Appelbaum FR, Ferrans VJ, et al (1981) Cardiotoxicity associated with high-dose cyclophosphamide therapy. Arch Int Med 141: 758

Hows JM, Menta A, Ward L, et al (1984) Comparison of Mesna with forced diuresis to prevent cyclophosphamide induced haemorrhagic cystitis in marrow transplantation: A prospective randomized study. Br J Cancer 50: 753

Meyers JD, Flournoy N, Thomas ED (1986) Risk factors for cytomegalovirus infection after human bone marrow transplantation. J Infect Dis 153: 478

Meyers JD, Shepp DH, Bowden RA, et al (1987) Viral infections in marrow transplant recipients. Progress in Bone Marrow Transplantation pp 545

Mills BA, Roberts RW (1979) Cyclophosphamide-induced cardiomyopathy. Cancer 43: 2223

Szeluga DJ, Stuart RK, Brookmeyer R, et al (1987) Nutritional support of bone marrow transplant recipients: A prospective, randomized clinical trial comparing total parenteral nutrition to an enteral feeding program. Cancer Res 47: 3309

Weiner RS, Bortin MM, Gale RP, et al (1986) Interstitial pneumonitis after bone marrow transplantation: Assessment of risk factors. Ann Int Med 104: 168

2. Acute Graft-versus-Host Disease

With a successful marrow transplant, the recipient's lymphohemopoietic cells are replaced by donor derived cells. Thus, in contrast to solid organ transplantation where the recipient's immune system remains in place and attempts at immunosuppression are aimed at preventing the reaction of recipient cells against the transplanted organ, the directions in marrow transplantation are basically reversed. Although a marrow transplant can also be rejected (see below), once engraftment has been achieved, the recipient's body is "invaded" by the donor derived immune system. Consequently, the potential complications are those of a reaction of donor derived cells against recipient tissue and organs. We have to assume that in all instances of marrow transplantation an interaction between donor and host cells (graft-vs-host reaction) takes place. However, it was noted in early experiments that syngeneic, i.e. genetically identical marrow, could be transferred to a pretreated recipient without any clinically recognizable adverse reaction. In contrast, when marrow from an allogeneic donor was used in clinical syndrome developed which was originally termed secondary disease. This syndrome, subsequently called graft-vs-host disease (GVHD), is manifested mostly in skin, liver, and intestinal tract, although other targets such as the conjunctivae can be involved as well (see Table 13).

Mechanisms of GVHD

Experimental studies soon suggested that the development of GVHD was closely related to the administration of immunocompetent lymphocytes from the marrow donor. There was evidence that increasing the number of lymphoid cells increased the likelihood, and shortened the time interval to the development of acute GVHD. Concurrent clinical observations indicated that a similar picture could develop after blood transfusions in immunologically deficient recipient's. Based on these and additional data, Billingham summarized the essential requirements for development of GVHD:

a) the graft must contain immunologically competent cells;
b) the recipient has to express relevant transplantation antigens that are not present in the donor, and consequently capable of immunologically stimulating donor cells;

c) the recipient has to be immunologically deficient, i.e. incapable of showing an immune response that would result in the destruction of transplanted or transfused donor cells.

Subsequent studies revealed differences in the potential of various lymphocyte populations to induce GVHD. This potential appeared to reside mostly in small lymphocytes, and was stronger in peripheral blood than in lymph nodes, spleen, or marrow cells. It was also shown that marrow cells, although incapable of directly triggering a graft-versus-host reaction, could differentiate into cells which were capable of doing so. By the mid 1970s' it was clear that T lymphocytes played a pivotal role in the initiation of GVHD. Studies in mice, rats, dogs, and nonhuman primates have shown that depletion of donor marrow T and possibly pre-T lymphocytes by conventional antisera, monoclonal antibodies, density gradients, or other methods may prevent or reduce the incidence of GVHD. There is evidence, however, albeit less compelling, that other factors are involved. Experimental studies suggest that host macrophages, and both host and donor natural killer cells may be involved. It has also been pointed out that the major target organs for acute GVHD are those that are particularly rich in dendritic cells, implying that antigen presenting cells of the recipient may be involved in the development of GVHD.

Another fact thought to be relevant to the development of GVHD is host contamination by bacteria. Studies in murine models have shown that lethally irradiated germfree animals given marrow grafts from germfree donors developed no GVHD as compared to a 100% fatality rate related to GVHD in control mice maintained in a conventional environment. The reasons for this are not entirely clear. Conceivably, donor derived immunocompetent cells crossreact with bacterial antigens which share antigenic determinants with recipient tissues. Consequently, in the absence of these organisms, a graft-vs-host reaction might be aborted, once the relevant recipient target cells have been eliminated, but might be propagated in the presence of the relevant organisms even after the immediate graft-vs-host reaction involving the recipient's tissue has run its course. Clinical studies in patients with aplastic anemia support this notion. Both in pediatric and adult patients, the incidence of GVHD was lower and survival superior in patients who were placed in a laminar air flow room and given nonabsorbable oral antibiotics.

The development of GVHD after transplantation is a very important event since clinical manifestations of this disease are associated with a high morbidity and mortality, to a large extent due to the fact that GVHD markedly impairs immunoreconstitution following transplantation. It was hypothesized that GVHD could be prevented and tolerance established by eliminating host reactive lymphocyte clones of donor origin by a mechanism termed "clonal deletion" or "clonal abortion". An effect of blocking factors had been proposed but could not be confirmed. More recent data indicate that suppressor cells may play a role. Extrapolation of experimental data ot the clinical situation is hampered by the fact that, until recently, most animal studies were carried out in major histocompatibility complex incompatible donor recipient combinations, whereas most clinical transplants use major histocompatibility complex (HLA) compatible donors, different from recipients only for minor (non-HLA) antigens. Experiments in rats given cyclosporine after transplantation revealed the presence of nonspecific suppressor cells early after transplant. Subsequently, these were replaced by suppressor cells specific for the host histocompatibility type. There was no evidence for clonal deletion. Experiments in dogs using haploidentical marrow grafts and post grafting immunosuppression with methotrexate and cyclosporine revealed different results. Dogs that did not develop GVHD had circulating host specific suppressor cells. In vitro experiments, however, showed that even after removal of suppressor cells, chimera cells failed to respond to host cells, suggesting a role for clonal abortion or deletion, possibly mediated by suppressor cells.

Extensive studies have been carried out in patients given HLA identical marrow graft, usually followed by post-grafting immunosuppression with methotrexate. By definition, lymphocytes from the marrow donor were unresponsive to host cells. However, donor derived lymphocytes in the transplant recipient, after transplantation, showed proliferation in mixed leukocyte culture against host cells in one third of patients with chronic GVHD. Nonspecific suppressor cells, i.e. lymphocytes that suppress the proliferation of donor cells against cells from unrelated controls, were generally absent early after transplantation in patients both with and without GVHD, as well as in long term survivors without GVHD. Nonspecific suppressor cells were, however, present in many patients with chronic GVHD. Lymphocytes obtained from longterm healthy survivors without GVHD specifically suppressed the response of donor lymphocytes to trinitrophenol modified host cells. Studies are currently underway in patients given cyclosporine after transplantation in an attempt to determine whether a different mechanism might be involved in these patients. There is evidence from transplant studies in rats that this may indeed be the case. Until more detailed study results become available, one must conclude, at the present time, that nonspecific suppressor cells are associated with the presence of GVHD especially in its chronic form, whereas specific suppressor cells, possibly by mediating clonal abortion, result in the development of transplantation tolerance.

GVHD After Autologous Transplants

GVHD by definition should occur only if histocompatibility differences exist between marrow donor and recipient. However, it has been noted that occasionally patients given syngeneic or autologous grafts develop a syndrome which is clinically, histologically, and by laboratory parameters indistinguishable from GVHD after allogeneic transplantation. The reasons for this are not entirely clear. Conceivably the reaction is due to immunological dysregulation with the appearance of autoreactive cells. It has also been postulated that host cells may be modified by the conditioning regimen or by viral infections, and those changes may be sensed as "non-self" by the transplanted cells, thus leading to a pseudo graft-vs-host reaction. If this syndrome develops, treatment is the same as that described below for allogeneic GVHD.

Table 13. Targets of Acute GVHD

Skin
Liver
Intestinal Tract
Conjunctivae
Airways (?)
Exocrine glands (?)

Clinical Features of GVHD

Acute GVHD in a human patient usually develops within 2–10 weeks of marrow transplantation. The main target organs are listed in Table 13. Figure 3 summarizes the clinical grading. There is no universal agreement as to how GVHD should best be graded. Although the criteria originally proposed by the Seattle group continue to form the basis of all grading systems, some modifications appear indicated. Hepatic enzyme abnormalities in addition to elevated bilirubin should be considered. Also, fever and fluid retention clearly are part of hyperacute GVHD seen with HLA-nonidentical transplants and in patients not given

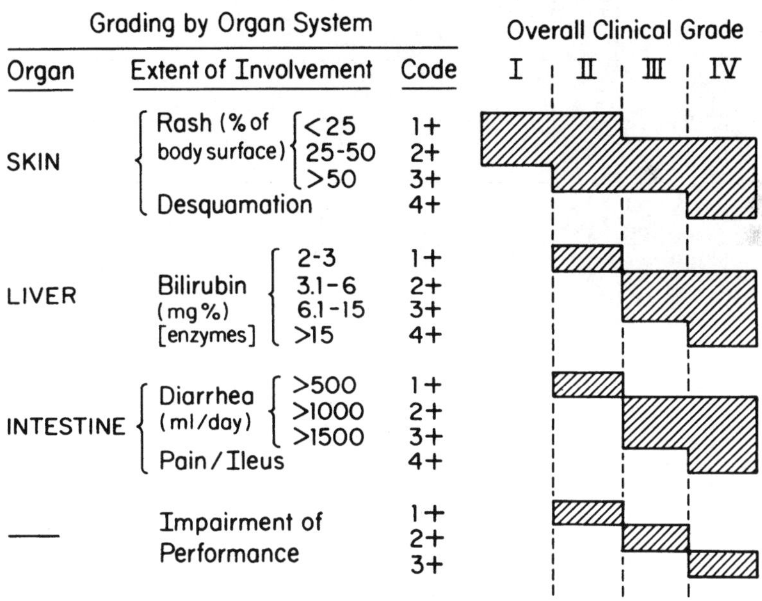

Fig. 3. Clinical grading of acute GVHD. The left panel of the figure summarizes the grading by organ system; the right panel shows the overall clinical grade. With grade I, only the skin can be involved. With more extensive involvement of the skin or involvement of liver and intestinal tract and impairment of the clinical performance status, either alone or in any combination, the severity grade advances from II to IV. (Reprinted with permission from H. J. Deeg et al, "Graft-versus-host disease: Pathophysiological and clinical aspects", Ann. Rev. Med. 1984, 35:11–24)

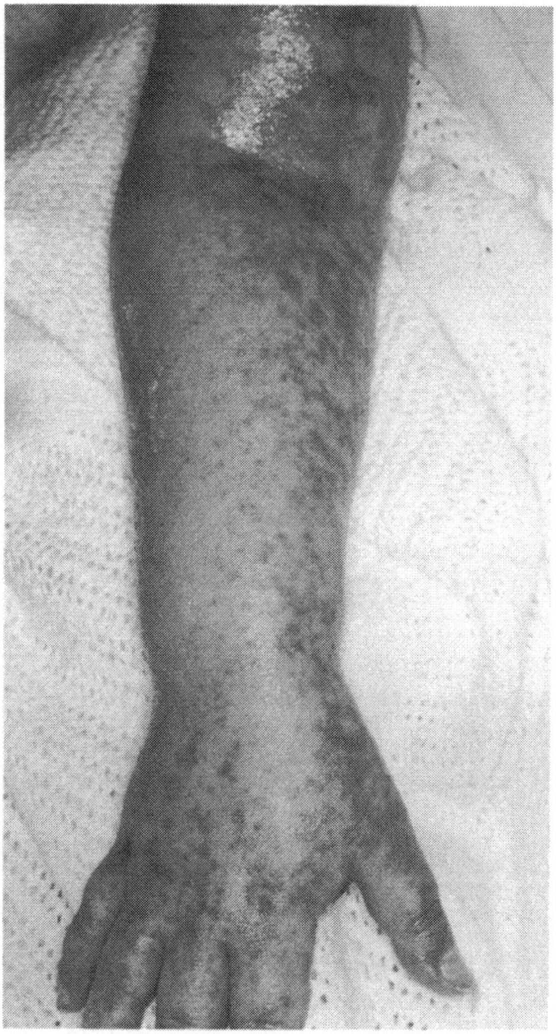

Fig. 4. Acute GVHD of the skin with diffuse erythema and superimposed maculopapular eruption and associated edema of the dermis (courtesy of H. M. Shulman, M.D.)

post grafting immunosuppression. The onset of acute GVHD is usually marked by a maculo-papular rash involving face, palms and soles, subsequently spreading and possibly involving the entire body (Fig. 4). It can lead to formation of bullae, and have the appearance of a total body burn. Concurrently or subsequently, the bilirubin may rise along with an elevation of serum alkaline phosphatase and aspartate aminotransferase. There may also be nausea and vomiting along with watery or bloody diarrhea, and abdominal pain. Some diagnostic procedures are listed in Table 14. The radiographical appearance of the intestinal tract is illustrated by Figure 5. The histological alterations have been described elsewhere. Although only a rare patient will die from causes *directly* related to acute GVHD, 5–10% of patients will succumb to associated complications. Infections are frequent during the first 3–4 months and are described in detail below.

Table 14. Diagnosis of Acute GVHD

Clinical Picture (Skin, Liver, Intestinal Tract)
Skin Biopsy
Rectal Biopsy
Chemistry Survey
Radiograph of the Abdomen
(Gastric or Duodenal Biopsy)
(Liver Biopsy)

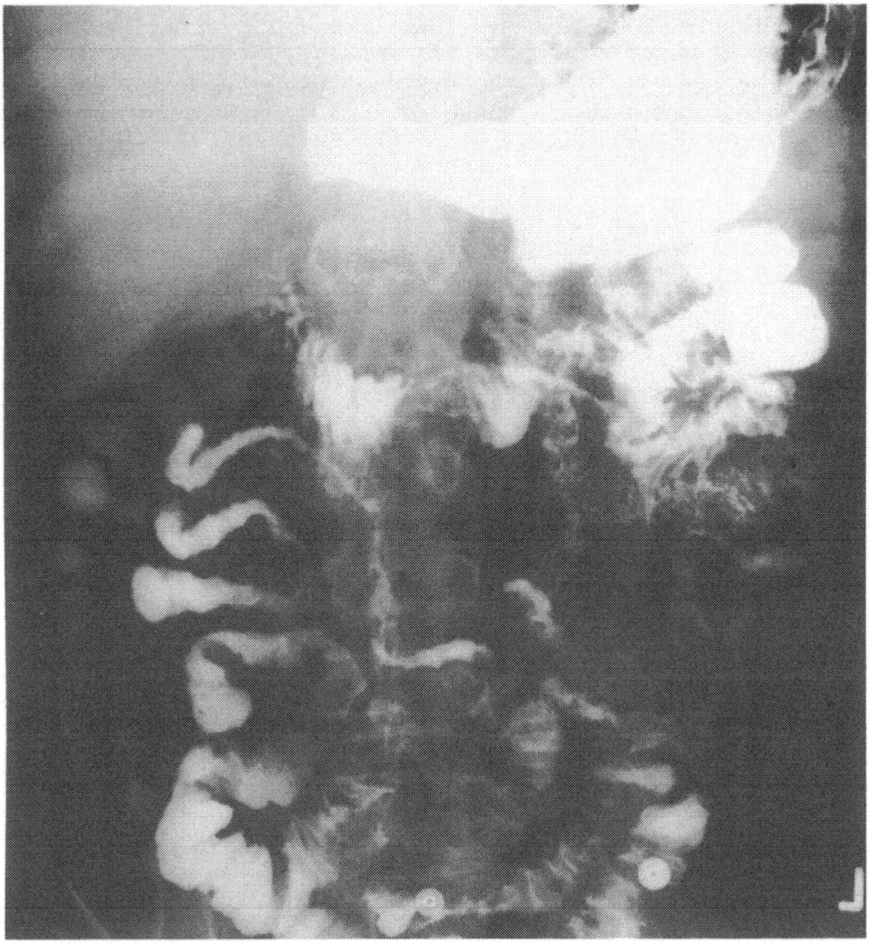

Fig. 5. Barium contrast radiograph of stomach and small bowel of a patient with acute GVHD. Stomach and duodenum are normal in appearance. There is edema of the bowel wall from mid-jejunum to terminal ileum with luminal narrowing, thumbprinting, and separation of adjacent loops (courtesy of G. McDonald, M.D.)

Table 15. Timing of GVHD Prophylaxis

* Donor treatment before marrow aspiration
* Marrow manipulation in vitro
– opsonization
– T-cell elimination
* Recipient treatment
– before marrow transplant
– after marrow transplant

Prevention of GVHD With Drugs

From the earlier discussion it is clear that several options for GVHD prevention are available. These are schematically summarized in Table 15. Conceivably, one could treat the marrow, which is to be transplanted, while it is still residing in the prospective marrow donor. Studies in rodent models suggest that antisera or monoclonal antibodies directed at T lymphocytes or at large granular lymphocytes may have a beneficial effect on the development of GVHD in the prospective recipient. Only one clinical study has been reported to date. Jacobs and coworkers treated prospective marrow donors with cyclosporine for 2 weeks prior to marrow aspiration and transplantation into the recipient. In this small uncontrolled study no advantage to this approach was noted.

Based on a large body of animal data, most clinical studies have used post transplantation treatment of the recipient with immunosuppressive agents. Until recently the two most widely applied regimens involved small doses of methotrexate or cyclophosphamide given intermittently for approximately three months after transplantation. This approach resulted in a 35–50% incidence of acute GVHD. In the late 1970s' cyclosporine became available, and was tested in numerous studies. Despite initial enthusiasm about this drug and noncontrolled studies suggesting that acute GVHD could be prevented almost completely, subsequent investigations resulted in a more realistic assessment. Cyclosporine was usually given on a daily basis starting one day before marrow infusion and continued for variable periods of time after transplantation, generally ranging from 3–12 months. With the oral preparation of the drug, the doses ranged from 10–25 mg/kg, generally around 12 mg/kg/d. Three randomized studies have been reported comparing methotrexate with cyclosporine in patients with various hematologic malignancies. The incidence of acute GVHD of grades II–IV ranged from 19–57% in patients given methotrexate, and from 40–56% in patients given cyclosporine. Overall there was no significant difference or advantage for either one of the drugs above. These results raised again the question as to whether any one of these agents might have a beneficial effect. This question appeared to be particularly important since both agents had significant associated toxicity.

A study by Lazarus and coworkers revealed a comparable incidence of GVHD for patients given methotrexate as compared to those given no postgrafting prophylaxis. Similarly, a study reported from the Dana Farber Cancer Center in Boston comparing, in sequential fashion, a standard course of methotrexate as described above with a short course of methotrexate, given on days 1 to 6, found a comparable (rather high) incidence of GVHD, in the range of 60–70%. Studies carried out at the Fred Hutchinson Cancer Research Center in Seattle showed that patients less than 30 years of age, and transplanted from HLA identical donors, had a 25% incidence of acute GVHD with a standard course of methotrexate, 61% with a short course of methotrexate and 100% without post grafting immunosuppression. These results, along with anecdotal data, strongly suggest that postgrafting immunosuppression is effective and that no allogeneic transplant without GVHD prophylaxis should be carried out.

The usefulness of postgrafting immunosuppression is further substantiated by recent trials using combinations of drugs. A study reported from the University of Minnesota using a combination of methotrexate, prednisone, and antithymocyte globulin (ATG) showed an incidence of acute GVHD of 21% compared to 48% in a control group given methotrexate only. Two studies from Seattle comparing cyclosporine and methotrexate given alone as compared to a combination of cyclosporine plus methotrexate resulted in a reduction of acute GVHD of grades II–IV from 54% to 33% and 53% to 18% respectively. Similarly, a study at City of Hope comparing methotrexate plus prednisone and cyclosporine plus prednisone found an incidence of acute GVHD of 28% in patients given the cyclosporine combination. A study reported from Johns Hopkins University in Baltimore, comparing cyclosporine plus prednisone to cyclophosphamide plus prednisone found a significant reduction of GVHD from 68% to 32% using the cyclosporine combination. A 30% incidence of acute GVHD was also reported with a cyclosporine/prednisone combination used at Ohio State University. Since very few, or no engraftment failures have been observed with these regimens, combinations of cyclosporine with methotrexate or cyclosporine with prednisone appear to be the best currently available GVHD prophylactic regimens.

Prevention of GVHD by T-Cell Depletion of Donor Marrow

Following the recognition in animal models that T lymphocytes played an essential role in the initiation of GVHD, studies were carried out to test this hypothesis. Indeed, it could be shown that mice transplanted across major histocompatibility barriers with T lymphocyte depleted marrow did not develop GVHD, and reconstituted to become completely immunocompetent chimeras. Similar, although less comprehensive, studies were reported in dogs and monkeys. Based on that information clinical trials were initiated. Methods used for T-cell depletion are listed in Table 11. Rodt and coworkers used a heteroantiserum directed at human lymphocytes to incubate donor bone marrow cells before infusion into the recipient. No complement source was added in the hope that opsonization of T lymphocytes would result in their rapid removal by the reticuloendothelial system of the recipient. They treated 20 patients with this approach, and only six developed signs of GVHD. It was of note, however, that 2 patients failed to achieve engraftment.

With the arrival of monoclonal antibodies directed at specific subpopulations of human cells, individual antibodies, or combinations thereof, have been used to manipulate marrow. Mouse monoclonal antibodies with pan-T specificity, or with specificities directed at subpopulations of T cells, have generally been used in conjunction with rabbit complement to eliminate the relevant cells in vitro before infusion into the recipient. This approach has been used for both HLA indentical and nonidentical transplants. Studies are too numerous to be listed individually, but results can be summarized as follows: effective depletion of T lymphocytes results in a reduced incidence of acute GVHD. The incidence of chronic GVHD remains to be determined. Concurrently with the reduction of GVHD, however, investigators noted problems wiht sustained engraftment. This problem was even more prominent with histoincompatible transplants, resulting in failure of sustained engraftment in as many as 60% of recipients given haplotype mismatched marrow. Some investigators argue that failure of engraftment was only due to insufficient immunosuppression of the recipient. Conceivably, the complete or partial elimination of immunocompetent donor T lymphocytes not only eliminated the effector cells of GVHD, but also of a anti-host reactivity necessary for optimum engraftment. Hence, the effect otherwise mediated by donor T lymphocytes would have to be achieved by other means, i.e. additional immunosuppression of the recipient. If this speculation is correct, however, it would also point the way towards a more specific approach, i.e. a more selective inhibition of host cells, thereby avoiding increased toxicity otherwise associated with brader and more aggressive immunosuppression of the recipient. In those patients who did achieve engraftment, one encouraging observation was that the immunoreconstitution proceeded at a rate comparable to that seen in patients given unmanipulated normal bone marrow. For some patient populations, such as children with SCID, T cell depleted marrow transplantation represents at present the treatment of choice. For patients with other disorders, especially with non-malignant hemopoietic diseases such as severe aplastic anemia, the risk of non-engraftment has to be weighed against that of developing GVHD.

In part due to the concern about unreliability of complement sources, numerous investigators have attempted to find means of T cell elemination that did not depend upon complement. Pioneered by Reisner and coworkers a method combining the use of soybean agglutination and rosette formation with sheep red blood cells was used effectively at Sloan Kettering Memorial Cancer Center, to eliminate T cells from donor marrow, thereby preventing the development of GVHD in the recipients. The disadvantage of this method is the time required for its' completion. Other methods, at the present time, use for example monoclonal antibodies coupled to magnetic beads. The antibodies will attach to the relevant cells which in turn are removed by passage through a strong magnetic field. Another approach is the coupling of monoclonal antibodies to immunotoxins such as ricin A chain. Following the binding of the antibody to the relevant cell, the ricin will enter the cell and destroy it. Another approach involves the use of density gradients. This was originally proposed by Dicke and colleagues using albumin gradients, which resulted in a good separation of immunocompetent and hemopoietic stem cells in animal models. More recently several investigators have used successfully discontinuous percoll gradients to enrich for hemopoietic stem cells. The method of counter flow elutriation, basically a more sophisticated modification of the gradient technique uses different centrifuge speeds (rather than different densities) to separate different cell populations from each other. Several centers in Europe and in the United States have now reported very encouraging results with this method. Contrary to some of the studies using monoclonal antibody and complement, failure of engraftment did not appear to be a problem with marrow obtained by counterflow elutriation. Other efforts have been with chemoseparation using agents such as methylprednisone, for preincubation of donor marrow. Although quite promising in rodent models, preliminary clincal data have been disappointing.

Of note is the development of rat antihuman monoclonal antibodies, which activate human complement sufficiently to destroy the relevant cells. The most widely used antibody is campath 1, a broadly reactive antibody which recognizes the majority of human T cells, B cells, and some NK cells. At least 280 transplants from HLA identical donors using this approach have been reported. Preliminary analysis indicates that only 7% of these patients developed significant acute GVHD. However, similar to other studies using monoclonal antibodies, 16% of patients failed to achieve sustained engraftment.

Another disturbing finding in studies with campath 1 was the fact that 40% (in one study as many as 70%) of patients with chronic myelogenous leukemia had recurrence of their disease. In retrospect this may not be surprising. Studies in rodent models have shown that animals with leukemia that develop GVHD have a lower relapse rate of leukemia than recipients without GVHD. This effect has been termed graft-vs-leukemia reaction. More recently several analyses of clinical marrow transplant trials have also shown that patients with GVHD have a better chance of remaining in remission than patients without GVHD. Since GVHD is initiated by donor T lymphocytes it is thought that the graft-vs-leukemia effect is also mediated by this cell population. In mice this has indeed been shown to be the case, although it has been speculated that different T cell populations are involved or that the effects are dose (T cell number) depentent. Therefore, the removal of T cells from the marrow may prevent not only GVHD but conceivably also the "byproduct", a graft-vs-leukemia effect. Several other studies on T cell depletion suggest that T cell depletion may increase the risk for leukemia recurrence in other subtypes of leukemia as well. At the present time, investigations are under way to determine whether this problem can be overcome by partial or by more selective T cell depletion.

The Effect of a Germ-Free Environment on GVHD

Finally, the approach of transplanting patients in a germfree environment after skin and gastrointestinal decontamination is rather attractive, although logistically quite involved and not inexpensive. It is, furthermore, of note that to date positive results have been reported only in patients with nonmalignant diseases, i.e. patients conditioned with chemotherapy alone, rather than regimens including the use of TBI. Presumably, patients given only chemotherapy had less gastrointestinal toxicity and were able to comply with the administration of oral nonabsorbable antibiotics, resulting in sufficient decontamination to have an impact on the development of GVHD. In patients given TBI, presumably, compliance was poor, decontamination was less successful, and consequently, GVHD developed. This observation would be entirely in agreement with the hypothesis that normally occurring organisms in the intestinal tract or on the skin might play an important bystander role in the development of GVHD.

Treatment of GVHD

Agents used experimentally or clinically for prophylaxis or treatment of GVHD are listed in Table 16. All approaches are immunosuppressive. GVHD itself also has an immunosuppressive effect. Thus, if, despite prophylaxis GVHD develops, a profound state of immunosuppression is reached. However, any available treatment again consists of additional immunosuppression in the form of glucocorticoids, ATG, cyclosporine, or monoclonal antibody. With all modalities, responses in the range of 30% have been achieved. Combinations of various agents such as ATG and cyclosporine in patients given methotrexate prophylaxis appear to be somewhat more effective. With improved results using cyclosporine-containing prophylactic regimens, fewer patients require additional treatment, and those who do appear to respond better to secondary therapy than patients on methotrexate prophylaxis. As additional agents are being used for prophylaxis, the choices of a therapeutic regimen become more limited. It is possible, however, to increase the dose of cyclosporine (as long as renal function permits) or to administer the same monoclonal antibody that had been used previously to treat the bone marrow in vitro. Trials are underway with antibodies directed at the interleukin 2 receptor, or with antibodies coupled to immunotoxin. Very encouraging experimental data have also been reported with the use of thalidomide.

Table 16. Agents Used for Prevention and Treatment of GVHD

Methotrexate	L-Asparaginase
Azathioprine	Glucocorticoids
6 Mercaptopurine	Cyclosporine
2-Deoxycoformicin	Antithymocyte globulin (ATG)
Cyclophosphamide	Monoclonal antibodies
Procarbazine	4-Hydroperoxycyclophosphamide
Cytosine arabinoside	Thalidomide
Chlorambucil	

References

Bortin MM (1987) Factors influencing the risk of acute graft-vs-host disease in man. Progress in Bone Marrow Transplantation R P Gale and R Champlin (eds) Alan R Liss, Inc., New York pp 243

Deeg HJ, Doney K, Sullivan KM, Witherspoon RP, Appelbaum FR, Storb R (1987) Prevention and treatment of graft-versus-host disease (GVHD) with drugs. Progress in Bone Marrow Transplantation, Alan R Liss, Inc., R P Gale and R Champlin (eds) pp 265

Deeg HJ. Storb R (1984) Graft-versus-host disease: pathophysiological and clinical aspects. Ann Rev Med 35: 11

Forman SJ, Blume KG, Krance RA, Miner PJ, Metter GE, Hill LR, O'Donnell MR, Nademanee AP, Snyder DS (1987) A prospective randomized study of acute graft-v-host-disease in 107 patients with leukemia: methotrexate/prednisone v cyclosporine A/prednisone. Transplant Proc 19: 2605

Glucksberg H, Storb R, Fefer A, Buckner CD, Neiman PE, Clift RA, Lerner KG, Thomas ED (1974) Clinical manifestations of graft-versus-host disease in human recipients of marrow from HL-A-matched sibling donors. Transplantation 18: 295

Grebe SC, Streilein JW (1976) Graft-versus-host reactions. A review. Adv Immunol 22: 119

Hale G, Bright S, Chumbley G, Hoang T, Metcalf D, Munro AJ, Waldmann H (1983) Removal of T cells from bone marrow for transplantation: A monoclonal antilymphocyte antibody that fixes human complement. Blood 62: 873

Herve P, Cahn JY, Flesch M, Plouvier E, Racadot E, Noir A, Couteret G, Goldstein G, Bernard A, Lenys R, Bresson JL, Leconte des Floris R, Peters A (1987) Successful graft-versus-host disease prevention without graft failure in 32 HLA-identical allogeneic bone marrow transplantations with marrow depleted of T cells by monoclonal antibodies and complement. Blood 69: 338

Kernan NA, Collins NH, Juliano L, Cartagena T, Dupont B, O'Reilly R (1986) Clonable T lymphocytes in T cell-depleted bone marrow transplant correlate with development of graft-v-host disease. Blood 68: 770

Korngold R, Sprent J (1978) Lethal graft-versus-host disease after bone marrow transplantation across minor histocompatibility barriers in mice. Prevention by removing mature T cells from marrow. J Exp Med 148: 1687

Lazarus HM, Coccia PF, Herzig RH, Graham-Pole J, Gross S, Strandjord S, Gordon E, Cheung NKV, Warkentin PI, Spitzer TR, Warm SE (1984) Incidence of acute graft-versus-host disease with and without methotrexate prophylaxis in allogeneic bone marrow transplant patients. Blood 64: 215

Mitsuyasu RT, Champlin RE, Gale RP, Ho WG, Lenarsky C, Winston D, Selch M, Elashoff R, Giorgi JV, Wells J, Terasaki P, Billing R, Feig S (1986) Treatment of donor bone marrow with monoclonal anti T-cell antibody and complement for the prevention of graft-versus-host disease. A prospective, randomized, double-blind trial. Ann Int Med 105: 20

Prentice HG, Brenner MK, Grob JP, Janossy G, Wimperis J, Hoffbrand AV, Gilmore M, Thomas AE, Hancock J, Pattinson JK, Bell N, Skeggs D (1987) Bone marrow transplantation in the treatment of acute leukaemia in first remission using T-lymphocyte depleted marrow from HLA identical sibling donors. Progress in Bone Marrow Transplantation R. P. Gale and R. Champlin (eds) Alan R Liss, Inc., pp 337

Ramsay NK, Kersey JH, Robison LL, McGlave PB, Woods WG, Krivit W, Kim TH, Goldman AI, Nesbit Jr, ME (1982) A randomized study of the prevention of acute graft-versus-host disease. N Eng J Med 306: 392

Rappeport J, Mihm M, Reinherz E, Lopansri S, Parkman R (1979) Acute graft-versus-host disease in recipients of bone-marrow transplants from identical twin donors. The Lancet II 717

Ringden O, Nilsson B (1985) Death by graft-versus-host disease associated with HLA mismatch, high recipient age, low marrow cell dose, and splenectomy, Transplantation 40: 39

Sale GE, Shulman HM (1984) The pathology of bone marrow transplantation. Masson Publishing USA, Inc., New York

Santos GW, Hess AD, Vogelsang GB (1985) Graft-versus-host reactions and disease. Immunol Rev 88: 169

Tsoi MS (1982) Immunological mechanisms of graft-versus-host-disease in man. Transplantation 33: 459

Storb R, Deeg JH, Whitehead J, Appelbaum F, Beatty P, Bensinger W, Buckner D, Clift R, Doney K, Farewell V, Hansen J, Hill R, Lum L, Martin P, McGuffin R, Sanders J, Stewart P, Sullivan K, Witherspoon R, Yee G, Thomas ED (1986) Methotrexate and cyclosporine compared with cyclosporine alone for prophylaxis of acute graft versus host disease after marrow transplantation for leukemia. N Eng J Med 314: 729

Storb R, Prentice RL, Buckner CD, Clift RA, Appelbaum F, Deeg HJ, Doney K, Hansen JA, Mason M, Sanders JE, Singer J, Sullivan KM, Witherspoon RP, Thomas ED (1983) Graft-versus-host disease and survival in patients with aplastic anemia treated by marrow grafts from HLA-identical siblings. Beneficial effect of a protective environment. N Eng J of Med 308: 302

Vogelsang GB, Hess AD, Berkman AW, Tutschka PJ, Farmer ER, Converse PJ, (1985) An in vitro predictive test for graft-versus-host disease in patients with genotypic HLA-identical bone marrow transplants. N. Eng J Med 313: 645

Vossen JM, Heidt PJ, Guiot HFL, Dooren LJ (1981) Prevention of acute graft versus host disease in clinical bone marrow transplantation: complete versus selective intestinal decontamination. S. Sasaki et al. (eds) Recent Advances in Germfree Research. pp 573, Tokai University Press

de Witte T, Hoogenhout J, de Pauw B, Holdrinet R, Janssen J, Wessels J, van Daal W, Hustinx T, Haanen C (1986) Depletion of donor lymphocytes by counterflow centrifugation successfully prevents acute graft-versus-host disease in matched allogeneic marrow transplantation. Blood 67: 1302

3. Marrow Graft Failure

To achieve sustained marrow engraftment, immunosuppressive therapy must be given to suppress the patient's own immune system and to allow donor-derived cells to replace the patient's lymphohemopoietic system. Under controlled experimental conditions it is possible to differentiate between graft rejection due to preceding sensitization, and failure of sustained engraftment in a nonsensitized recipient on the basis of genetic (hybrid, allogeneic) resistance. It is more difficult to separate these two mechanisms in man. However, both with and without sensitization graft failure can manifest itself either as primary engraftment failure or as initial engraftment followed by loss of the graft. This may or may not be associated with reappearance of recipient cells. Tests for documentation of donor cell engraftment are listed in Table 17. In some instances transplant recipients become "mixed chimeras", i.e. show coexistence of normal donor and host cells for prolonged periods of time (possibly indefinitely). The mechanisms involved are incompletely understood; however, at least four situations in which graft failure occurs can be differentiated:

a) In the presensitized patient given HLA identical unmanipulated marrow
b) In the patient transplanted with histoincompatible marrow
c) In the patient transplanted with T cell depleted marrow
d) In the patient transplanted with autologous marrow

The Presensitized Patient

Animal studies predict that a transplant recipient given transfusions before transplantation will be at increased risk of not accepting, i.e. rejecting a marrow graft

Table 17. Documentation of Engraftment of Donor Cells

Cytogenetic Analysis	– Sex Chromosome
	– Marker Chromosome (band)
Erythrocyte Typing	– Enzymes
	– Antigens
HLA Typing	
Complement Typing	
Immunoglobulin Allotyping	
Restriction Fragment Length Polymorphism (DNA)	

even from a histocompatible donor. This is indeed the case in clinical studies in patients with aplastic anemia. Patients who had been multiply transfused before marrow transplantation and who were conditioned with cyclophosphamide alone (without the use of TBI) in preparation for marrow transplantation for aplastic anemia had a probability of 30–60% of rejecting a graft from an HLA identical brother or sister, whereas only 5% of untransfused patients given the same conditioning regimen were found to reject their marrow graft. Results from animal studies suggested that graft rejection was due to sensitization of the recipient to minor histocompatibility antigens presumably shared between transfusion donor and marrow donor and not expressed on recipient cells. Exposure to those same antigens at the time of transplantation, therefore, represented a secondary immune response more difficult to suppress with conventional methods than a primary immune response encountered in nonsensitized patients.

Different transplant teams have used different approaches to overcome this problem. Based on studies in a dog model the Seattle group has added the infusion of viable peripheral blood leukocytes from the marrow donor to the marrow inoculum to achieve sustained engraftment in patients with aplastic anemia who were transfused prior to transplantation. This approach has been successful, and in the most recent trials has reduced the probability of rejection to approximately 5%, i.e. to a level not different from that seen in untransfused patients. As before, however, untransfused patients were given bone marrow only and no additional peripheral blood leukocytes. This difference is important since the infusion of donor leukocytes carries a higher risk for GVHD (especially chronic) than observed with marrow alone. Nevertheless, this approach appears to be justified since only approximately 25% of patients who reject their graft will survive as compared to 75% of patients achieving sustained engraftment. Recent data indicate that in pediatric patients (< 17 years) there may be a rather low risk of graft rejection even in transfused patients, and consequently buffy coat cells should probably be omitted. Other transplant teams have elected to overcome sensitization by increased immunosuppression, usually in the form of drugs or irradiation. Thus, the use of 300 cGy of TBI, or 750 cGy of total lymphoid irradiation (i.e. an approach similar to that used for the treatment of Hodgkin's disease, although to a lower total dose), or in a modified form given as thoraco-abdominal irradiation in addition to cyclosphosphamide, were successful in overcoming rejection. There is concern about the long-term effects of irradiation in patients with a nonmalignant disease, especially in children. Only further observations will allow us to determine whether longterm effects are acceptable. Alternatives include the use of a combination of cyclophosphamide and procarbazine, or antithymocyte globulin shown to be effective in small numbers of patients. Conceivably the use of monoclonal antibodies, in addition to cyclophosphamide, might yield similar results in the future.

From a practical point of view, these studies indicate that ideally a patient with aplastic anemia should be transplanted while still untransfused. Therefore, the physician who evaluates such a patient initially should be aware of these data, and assuming a potential marrow donor is available, should consider the possibility of a marrow transplant early on. A transplant center should be contacted immediately for consultation and recommendations in regards to the timing of transfusions. Only if the patient is actively bleeding, or requires surgery or some other intervention, should platelet transfusions be given before the situation can be assessed completely. Clinical data suggest that there may be a "window" of approximately 48–72 hours prior to the initiation of the conditioning regimen for transplantation during which transfusions can be given to the patient without jeopardizing the subsequent marrow graft.

Recent experiments suggest that it may be possible, in the future, to transfuse a patient without the risk of sensitization. Studies in dogs have shown that irradiation of blood (from the marrow donor) with ultraviolet light prior to transfusion abrogates the blood's sensitizing ability, and dogs so treated achieve sustained engraftment just as dogs who have never been transfused. Similarly, dogs given ultraviolet-irradiated platelets from histoincompatible donors are at a significantly lower risk of becoming sensitized and refractory to platelet transfusions than dogs given untreated platelets. There are also preliminary clinical data to suggest that aggressive leukocyte depletion of the transfusion product substantially reduces the risk of inducing sensitization. It appears that leukocytes with antigen presenting ability, such as monocytes, or more likely dendritic cells, are responsible for sensitization.

Pretransplant transfusions in patients with lymphohemopoietic malignancies are apparently not associated with an increased risk of marrow graft rejection. Presumably this is due to the more aggressive cytotoxic therapy, generally involving the use of TBI, that is usually employed to prepare these patients for transplantation. Furthermore, in these patients transfusions are generally required because of chemotherapy-induced myelosuppression. Conceivably this chemotherapy also has immunosuppressive effects, thus preventing the patient's immune system from responding to the alloantigenic challenge.

Histoincompatible Transplants

Except in patients with severe aplastic anemia, marrow graft rejection or failure of engraftment has generally not been a problem with HLA identical marrow grafts. More recently, however, as more histoincompatible transplants have been carried out, evidence has accumulated that even doses of 850–1500 cGy of TBI may be insufficient to suppress the recipient's immunresponse against major histocompatibility antigens. Dependent upon the degree of mismatch, as many as 15% of patients have shown failure of sustained engraftment, or incomplete hemopoietic reconstitution by donor cells.

As described above, graft failure can occur either in the form of primary failure of engraftment, or with initial evidence of engraftment followed by graft loss. In some respects, these observations resemble those made in animals, especially mice and dogs, showing the phenomenon of genetic resistance. This term generally refers to failure of sustained engraftment of histoincompatible marrow in a setting where major histocompatibility complex matched marrow easily engrafts. Regardless of the mechanism involved, major histocompatibility barriers do represent a problem. Since patients given histoincompatible grafts are more likely to develop GVHD and to have more severe manifestations of GVHD than patients transplanted with HLA identical marrow, they represent a main target group for aggressive attempts at GVHD prevention. Consequently T cell depletion is being tested widely in these patients. As will be seen, however, T cell depletion further aggravates the problem of resistance. So far, approaches to histoincompatible grafts have included increased doses of TBI, the addition of chemotherapy such as cytosine arabinoside to regimens consisting of cyclophosphamide and TBI, or the use of monoclonal antibodies and ATG. Interesting results have been obtained in a canine model with the infusion of monoclonal antibodies directed at class II histocompatibility antigens or at radiation resistant recipient cells in addition to a standard dose of TBI (9.2 Gy). This approach allowed for sustained engraftment in a large proportion of dogs, who with TBI alone almost uniformly fail to engraft. Initial clinical trails with an antibody directed at lymphocyte function antigen I (LFA I) suggest that such an approach might also be feasible and successful in patients.

T-Cell Depletion

Allogeneic marrow transplantation offers curative therapy for many patients suffering from acute or chronic leukemia, aplastic anemia, or congenital disorders. GVHD is one of the major complications associated with this approach even if the transplant is carried out from a genotypically HLA identical donor. Clinically significant acute GVHD has been observed in 35–50% of patients given methotrexate, cyclosporine, or cyclophosphamide as post grafting immunosuppressive prophylaxis. Among those patients who survive the acute phase, approximately 40% are expected to develop chronic GVHD. Even with regimens combining agents such as cyclosporine and methotrexate, or cyclosporine and methylprednisolone an incidence of acute GVHD in the range of approximately 30% in adult patients has been reported from several transplant centers. With HLA nonidentical transplants, dependent upon the degree of mismatch, as many as 60–90% of recipients are expected to develop significant acute GVHD. Since GVHD is associated with substantial morbidity and even mortality in those patients who are severely affected, it remains one of the most important complications after transplantation.

Studies in animal models have shown that mature donor T lymphocytes are responsible for causing GVHD after transplantation of allogeneic marrow or spleen cells. If the marrow is taken from animals that are devoid of mature T-Cells, or if T cells are removed, GVHD can be prevented. The same studies have shown that only very few T lymphocytes contained in the marrow or spleen cell inoculum can result in the development of GVHD even if the transplant is carried out in major histocompatibility complex identical animals i.e., in animals differing only for the so called minor antigens.

On this basis, removal of T lymphocytes from human marrow was attempted. The first attempts involved the use of a heteroantiserum generated in rabbits against human T lymphocytes. Subsequently, fractionation of marrow cells by means of agglutination with lectin, especially soybean agglutinin, and with sheep erythrocytes was achieved. Some studies have used physical methods. Most recent attempts, however, have focused on the use of monoclonal antibodies produced in mice or rats, and directed at specific surface molecules expressed on all human T lymphocytes, or on subpopulations of T cells. All studies involving monoclonal antibodies have shown that the use of an exogenous source of complement, or of the donor's own autologous complement is necessary for treatment success. Methods used to remove T lymphocytes in man are summarized in Table 11. The rationale for this approach is that only mature T cells induce GVHD. Thus, if mature cells are removed, those T cells developing from lymphohemopoietic stem cells, in a repetition of ontogeny, will differentiate and accept the new (patient) environment as "self", i.e. become tolerant.

In agreement with previous experimental data, T cell depletion of human marrow significantly reduces the incidence of acute GVHD. Chronic GVHD still occurs but the actual incidence remains to be determined. However, along with the very encouraging finding of reduced or absent acute GVHD several rather disturbing observations have been made. The first one was failure of sustained engraftment. Failure of engraftment or rejection in patients with a malignant disorder given TBI and an HLA identical marrow graft (without in vitro treatment) is highly unusual. A large series showed an incidence of only 0.1%. With T cell depleted marrow, graft failure has been observed in 15–35% of patients. The incidence was even higher in patients given HLA nonidentical transplants. It is thought that in this setting marrow graft rejection (or non-acceptance), unlike that observed in patients with aplastic anemia who were transfusion-sensitized prior to transplantation, is largely unrelated to pretransplant transfusions. Experimental results in mice and dogs have explained failure of engraftment in non-sensitized recipients on the basis of genetic resistance. Resistance is apparently mediated by antigens outside the major histocompatibility complex. Resistance can be overcome by more profound immunosuppression of the recipients or by measures directed more specifically at recipient cells involved in resistance. Regardless of the mechanism, these data imply that the presence of T lymphocytes in the marrow graft may have an immunosuppressive effect, either directly, or via the induction of a graft-vs-host reaction, which then might generate the milieu necessary for sustained engraftment. Alternatively, T lymphocytes may have an amplifier effect on transplanted hemopoietic stem cells, thus generating a growth advantage and leading to "take over" of the host. As a reaction to these observations, the trend has been to intensify immunosuppressive regimens used for conditioning. There is evidence that increased doses of TBI, or the addition of more cytotoxic drugs, or immunosuppressive agents such as antithymocyte globulin or monoclonal antibodies, might facilitate engraftment.

Graft failures have presented either as a priori non-engraftment, leaving the patient with marrow aplasia, or with initial engraftment and apparently normal hemopoiesis followed weeks to months later by a decline and frequently complete loss of donor cells. Attempts at second marrow transplants have almost uniformly been unsuccessful, either due to toxic side effects or to repeated failure of engraftment. It is important, therefore, to monitor not only a patient's blood counts, but also attempt to determine the origin of cells by cytogenetic analysis, by ABO blood type or by red cell antigen, or enzyme markers to ascertain that engraftment, indeed, was sustained.

Autologous Marrow Grafts

As outlined elsewhere, autologous transplantation, i.e. the use of the patient's own marrow for reconstitution of lymphohemopoietic function is being used with increasing frequency and success. There are basically three prerequisites for the feasibility of an autologous transplant:
- It must be possible to obtain sufficiently large numbers of hemopoietic stem cells capable of self replication and differentiation, and maintenance of viability of these cells.
- The stem cell preparation used for infusion should be free of clonogenic tumor cells.
- The patient's malignancy must be responsive to chemoradiotherapy usually given in superlethal doses in preparation for marrow transplantation. (This point, of course, applies not only to autologous, but also to allogeneic transplantation).

Stem cells obtained from the patient's bone marrow (or, for that purpose, from peripheral blood) have by necessity been exposed to chemotherapeutic regimens, irradiation or both given during initial treatment attempts of the patient. Thus, they have possibly suffered damage that might impair their ability to reconstitute hemopoietic function after transplantation. Also one might be left with cells that have suffered chromosomal damage but survive, and thus, could lead to the development of abnormal clones later on. There is, indeed, experimental and clinical evidence that the yield of stem cells, and possibly the quality, depends upon the time point following chemoradiotherapy at which stem cells are harvested. Dependent upon the agents used for chemotherapy, colony forming units are increased in peripheral blood at a certain time after institution of chemotherapy. Furthermore, there are experimental and clinical data indicating that the rate of hemopoietic recovery in the autologous setting depends upon the number of colony forming units (as an indirect assay for hemopoietic precursor cells). If recovery is slow, the time period of pancytopenia and transfusion dependence is prolonged, and this in turn means an increased risk of infections and transfusion related problems. These problems may make it necessary, for example, to obtain platelets from suitable selected donors, to provide single donor platelets from an HLA matched individual, or possibly from a family member sharing some of the patient's histocompatibility antigens.

To obtain the largest possible number of marrow cells is even more important when in vitro manipulation is being considered. The techniques available for autologous "marrow purging" are in principle those described for T cell depletion of allogeneic marrow. In addition, methods of chemoseparation, i.e. the use of chemotherapeutic agents, which preferentially damage or destroy malignant cells contained in the marrow have been developed for autologous transplantation. With these methods, summarized in Table 4, it may be difficult or even impossible to use in vitro hemopoietic assays to determine whether or not the manipulation has damaged the marrow. After treatment with 4-hydroperoxy-cyclophosphamide, for example, no colony forming units can be detected in in vitro systems. Nevertheless, marrow so treated (with a drug concentration determined empirically) is perfectly capable of reconstituting the patient's lymphohemopoietic system.

Finally, in many instances, bone marrow or peripheral blood stem cells harvested for autologous transplantation, must be cryopreserved in liquid nitrogen until later use. Cryopreservation can damage any cells, and stem cells in particular. Generally, the approach has been to obtain a large number of cells, such that a loss incurred during cryopreservation would be compensated for. It has been shown that even marrow cryopreserved for as long as 5–10 years can be used successfully for autologous reconstitution after marrow ablative therapy of patients.

However, despite all progress with autologous marrow transplantation there have been, and still are occasional patients who have incomplete reconstitution of hemopoiesis. Often these patients die with hemorrhage or infection. Most transplant teams have established a policy, that a second back-up marrow be stored and maintained unmanipulated to serve for rescue should the first transplant (with or without in vitro manipulation) be unsuccessful. There have been a few late marrow failures as long as six months after transplantation, but these seem to be rare.

Experience with peripheral blood stem cells is still too limited to allow for a projection as to what the long term outcome in these patients might be.

References

Blazar BR, Filipovich AH, Kersey JH, Uckun FM, Ramsay NKC, MacGlave PB, Vallera DA (1987) T-cell depletion of donor marrow grafts: Effects on graft-versus-host disease and engraftment. Progress in Bone Marrow Transplantation Gale RP and Champlin R (eds) Alan R Liss, Inc pp 381

Champlin RE, Feig SA, Gale RP (1984) Case problems in bone marrow transplantation. I. Graft failure in aplastic anemia: Its biology and treatment. Exp Hematol 12: 728

Deeg HJ, Self S, Storb R, Doney K, Appelbaum FR, Witherspoon RP, Sullivan KM, Sheehan K, Sanders J, Mickelson E, Thomas ED (1986) Decreased incidence of marrow graft rejection in patients with severe aplastic anemia: Changing impact of risk factors. Blood 68: 1363

Gorin NC, Douay L, Laporte JP, Lopez M, Mary JY, Najman A, Salmon C, Aegerter P, Stachowiak J, David R, Pene F, Kantor G, Deloux J, Duhamel E, van den Akker J, Gerota J, Parlier Y, Duhamel G (1986) Autologous bone marrow transplantation using marrow incubated with asta Z 7557 in adult leukemia. Blood 67: 1367

Hansen JA, Beatty PG, Anasetti C, Clift R, Martin PJ, Sanders J, Sullivan K, Buckner CD, Storb R, Thomas ED (1987) Treatment of leukemia by marrow transplantation from donors other than HLA genotypically identical siblings. Progress in Bone Marrow Transplantation Gale RP and Champlin R (eds), Alan R Liss, Inc pp 667

Juttner CA, To LB, Haylock DN, Branford A, Kimber RJ (1985) Circulating autologous stem cells collected in very early remission from acute non-lymphoblastic leukaemia produce prompt but incomplete haemopoietic reconstitution after high dose melphalan or supralethal chemoradiotherapy. Brit J Haematol 61: 739

Kernan NA, Flomenberg N, Dupont B, O'Reilly RJ (1987) Graft rejection in recipients of T-cell-depleted HLA-nonidentical marrow transplants for leukemia. Transplantation 43: 842

Martin PJ, Hansen JA, Buckner CD, Sanders JE, Deeg HJ, Stewart P, Appelbaum FR, Clift R, Fefer A, Witherspoon RP, Kennedy MS, Sullivan KM, Flournoy N, Storb R, Thomas ED (1985) Effects of in vitro depletion of T cells in HLA-identical allogeneic marrow grafts. Blood 66: 664

Ramsay NK, Kim TH, McGlave P, Goldman A, Nesbit, Jr. ME, Krivit W, Woods WG, Kersey JH (1983) Total lymphoid irradiation and cyclophosphamide conditioning prior to bone marrow transplantation for patients with severe aplastic anemia. Blood 62: 622
Storb R, Deeg HJ (1986) Failure of allogeneic canine marrow grafts after total-body irradiation. Allogeneic "Resistance" versus Transfusion-Induced Sensitization. Transplantation 42: 571

4. The Management of Infections

Overview

Virtually all marrow transplant recipients, regardless of marrow source, remain severely immunosuppressed some months after transplantation. In addition, immunologic recovery is gradual and variable, and certain processes (e.g., graft-vs-host disease, [GVHD]) and therapies (e.g., corticosteroids) are additionally immunosuppressive. Given this, it is hardly surprising that infections are nearly universal in the marrow transplant setting, and are a major cause of morbidity and mortality. In particular, GVHD and fatal infection are closely interrelated. However, infection is also a leading cause of non-malignant death in situations not associated with GVHD, i.e., autologous marrow transplants. Thus, proper management of infectious complications is mandatory to provide safer, more effective marrow transplantation.

As noted by other authors (see reviews by Bowden, Lum, Saral and Young and their colleagues), different phases of the marrow transplantation procedure are associated with varying deficiencies of the immune system. Infectious problems therefore may be considered according to the "phase" after transplantation in which they are most frequent, and are discussed accordingly.

Pre-Transplant Phase (Before Day 0). Patients are heterogeneous in terms of the clinical status of their immune systems pre-transplant. For example, acute leukemic patients undergoing transplantation during remission may be much less severely compromised than those in relapse, and chronic myelogenous leukemic patients in stable phase may be relatively normal.

Factors that may predispose the patient to infection after transplantation should be evaluated before the transplant sequence begins. Such factors include the presence of indwelling intravenous devices, organ obstruction, or a history of a previous infection that might be reactivated through immunosuppression. The latter pertains mainly to certain viruses, especially cytomegalovirus (CMV) and herpes simplex virus, but tuberculosis, aspergillosis, etc., should also be considered.

In addition, the pre-transplant evaluation should identify active infections, and treatment to resolve them should be completed before conditioning begins. In certain circumstances (e.g., aplastic anemia or relapsed acute leukemia), however, the resolution of infection may depend on the recovery from pancytopenia that will result only from a successful marrow transplant. In this case, appropriate anti-infective therapy and the transplant should be given concomitantly.

Generally speaking, truly prophylactic therapy is controversial and not usually recommended. However, therapies designed to suppress latent infections may be very helpful, as discussed below.

Immediate Post-Transplant Phase (Up to Day +30). During this period, profound neutropenia (less than $0.1 \times 10^9/L$) is invariably observed, and the problems arising are those generic to this situation, i.e., bacterial and fungal infections. The mucosal disruption that is variably produced by different conditioning regimens also predisposes to infections, especially to those caused by bowel flora (i.e., certain gram-negative aerobes). These factors, plus the effects of indwelling central venous catheters now commonly used, are felt to be of primary importance in the development of infections in this phase. Perhaps due to indwelling devices such as venous catheters, infection with gram-positive organisms, primarily coagulase-positive and coagulase-negative staphylococci, now exceed gram-negative aerobes as the most frequent source of bacterial infections at many institutions.

The clinical diagnosis and management of these infections is complicated both by the tissue damage of conditioning and by the absence of many of the classical signs of infection. Although fever is nearly universal with infections, it is nonspecific and may also be due to disease conditioning, other medications or transfusions. Despite severe infection, localized sites may show minimal (if any) clinical signs. For instance, perirectal infection may be marked only by pain and redness and not by swelling or abscess formation. While the lungs, perirectal area, skin, mouth and sinuses are the most common local sites of infection, virtually any site may be involved. Likewise, sepsis is often not associated with the usual stigmata of septic shock.

Because profound neutropenia minimizes the typical clinical signs of infection, and because inadequately-treated infection can be highly lethal in the marrow transplant setting, all febrile, neutropenic patients should be given immediate empiric broad-spectrum antimicrobial therapy. (It is important to note that this recommendation applies as well to neutropenic patients with other putative causes of fever, e.g., transfusions.) Empiric therapy usually consists of two or three antibiotics, including a semisynthetic penicillin and an aminoglycoside. The effective use of the latter should always be documented with serum assays. While antibiotic monotherapy with the third-generation cephalosporine ceftazidime, or with a broad-spectrum drug such as imipenemcilastatin, is attractive, it is not yet standard practice. Specific antistaphylococcal coverage with vancomycin is often added, especially since the use of indwelling intravenous catheters and related infections with *S. epidermidis* is so common. However, some investigators believe this policy is wasteful, since vancomycin is expensive, and these organisms are of a lesser virulence, readily cultured and treated. Perhaps most importantly, in choosing an empiric antibiotic regimen one should be aware of the patterns of infection in one's own institution.

For patients who respond to empiric antibiotics, therapy is usually continued until the neutrophil count exceeds $0.5 \times 10^9/L$, or somewhat longer if bacteremia was present. (As well, those patients with moderate or severe acute GVHD should also be continued on antibiotics.) For patients persistently febrile after 3–7 days of antimicrobial therapy, recommendations are more variable. Amphotericin B is often recommended empirically, based on the fact that the deep fungal infections that are common in this circumstance (usually *Candida* or *Aspergillus spp.*) are very difficult to diagnose antemortem; they must be treated early and vigorously to produce survival. However, this use of amphotericin B is controversial and other causes of persistent fever must also be considered, including resistant bacterial infection, drug fever, and indwelling central venous line infection.

Neutrophil transfusions are seldom used at present. However, they may be considered for patients who have suboptimal early responses to conventional antibiotics and who are at risk for prolonged neutropenia, or when the organisms appear resistant to available antibiotics. Although unproven, the use of more than a single neutrophil transfusion per day may be of greater benefit in desperate situations.

Many patients experience severe therapy-related mucositis shortly after the conditioning regimen is completed. Not only does mucositis predispose to certain bacterial infections as discussed above, but the reactivation of oral (or genital) herpes simplex infections is also common, and these can easily be confused with therapy-induced mucositis. Systemic acyclovir prophylaxis is very effective and should be given to all patients sero-positive for herpes simplex; if this is not done, acyclovir therapy should at least be administered to patients who develop herpetic infections. Topical antifungal agents such as clotrimazole may be useful in preventing oropharyngeal candidiasis. If severe mucosal candidiasis develops, low-dose amphotericin (i.e., 20 mg per day for 1–2 weeks) may be helpful and is only minimally toxic.

The use of multi-lumen indwelling central venous catheters has revolutionized the day-to-day management of transplant patients. However, these advances have been achieved at the cost of an increase of certain infections, e.g., those caused by gram-positive bacteria. Somewhat surprisingly, the routine removal of these lines during an infective episode is unnecessary unless any of the following conditions is present:

a) persistent infection (sepsis, or tunnel or exit-site infections) despite appropriate antimicrobial coverage;
b) fungal sepsis; or
c) clot at the catheter tip in the presence of sepsis.

In any event, these lines must be meticulously cared for by trained personnel-including the patient and family after discharge. Such catheters should always be considered as a source of infection or fever, and their use is an argument for the inclusion of vancomycin in primary empiric antimicrobial regimens.

Given the high morbidity and mortality associated with infections during neutropenia, they should be prevented whenever possible. Certain preventative measures, such as good personal hygiene (especially handwashing) and high-efficiency particulate air (HEPA) filtration, are important. On the other hand, neither prophylactic neutrophil transfusions nor prophylaxis against bacterial infections with co-trimoxazole before recovery of the neutrophil count are routinely recommended, due to the transmission of CMV infections and the emergence of resistant organisms, respectively. The use of a "total protective environment," including decontamination of the patient's skin and bowel mucosa and the use of laminar air flow (LAF) filtration, decreases infections but is very labor-intensive and expensive, and has not uniformly improved survival in controlled trials.

It is interesting to try to reconcile the seemingly contradictory observations that there is a high degree of immunosuppression produced by marrow transplant regimens, yet a relatively low infective death rate in the period before engraftment. In general, it is likely that several factors are responsible:

a) methods of infection prevention and treatment are now quite effective;
b) routine marrow transplantation in a patient with normal blood counts at the initiation is associated with a relatively brief period of neutropenia; and
c) some element of residual host immunity, or transfer of existing donor immunity, is likely.

Intermediate Post-Transplant Phase (Days +30 to +100). After neutrophil recovery, the bacterial and fungal infections discussed above usually improve, although they do not always resolve. (This finding may be related to functional defects of neutrophils, which can persist months after transplantation.) Moreover, severe humoral or cellular immunosuppression persists during and even beyond this period. Most significantly, acute GVHD often is either present before or may develop between days +30 and +100, requiring increased immunosuppressive therapy. Therefore, most of the serious infections seen during this phase are in patients with GVHD, reflecting the persistent deficiencies in neutrophil dysfunction, as well as in humoral and cell medicated immunity present with this GVHD. Frequently these infections involve the lungs, which also may be related to certain elements (especially total body irradiation) of conditioning regimens and a general impairment of mucociliary action. Interestingly, LAF facilities have been shown to reduce acute GVHD in patients with severe aplastic anemia who undergo marrow transplantation. This finding may be analogous to the decreased incidence of GVHD in gnotobiotic animals, suggesting that certain infections may play a role in triggering GVHD.

The lung infections mentioned above may be focal, and are often due to bacteria or fungi. Frequently, however, a diffuse interstitial pattern is noted radiographically. These are generally referred to as "interstitial pneumonias" and are often due to cytomegalovirus (CMV). As well, *Pneumocystis carinii*, adenovirus, herpes simplex virus and *Legionella pneumophila* are occasionally etiologic.

Effective prophylaxis may be administered to patients with such infections, with favorable results. For example, *P. carinii* has been largely prevented by co-trimoxazole prophylaxis. However, due to its myelosuppressive potential, co-trimoxazole should be started only after the neutrophils recover and blood counts must be monitored closely for depression. Co-trimoxazole may be given only for 2–3 days per week and is continued until some weeks after all immunosuppressives have been stopped. There is also evidence that interstitial pneumonitis due to CMV can be decreased either by the use of CMV-negative blood products in

CMV-seronegative donor-patient pairs or by the use of intravenous immunoglobulin with a high CMV titer. While the former is clearly of benefit, it is not clear how the various immunoglobulin preparations are best administered. Additional clinical trials are required to determine this. Moreover, the role of either of these measures in seropositive patients is speculative.

While the management of patients with interstitial pneumonitis is controversial, an aggressive approach to obtaining tissue is recommended. Specifically, bronchoscopy and bronchoalveolar lavage should be performed within the first few hours after presentation. Special rapid-diagnostic techniques, especially those for CMV, *L. pneumophila*, and *P. carinii* should be performed, and if these assays are non-diagnostic, an open lung biopsy should be arranged promptly. The alternative approach is to use broad-spectrum empiric therapy. Although the morbidity of the diagnostic procedures is avoided (at least initially) with this approach, empiric therapy may cause adverse drug interactions and toxicity due to multiple agents. Moreover, since there are potentially many organisms that must be dealt with, further empiric agents or a subsequent invasive diagnostic procedure in a weakened patient will be required if the response is unsatisfactory.

Other infections commonly noted during this period include sinusitis (due to either bacteria or fungi), cutaneous infection, or sepsis due to indwelling central venous catheter infections. Rarely, unusual parasitic organisms (such as toxoplasma) may be noted during this period. As with the interstitial pneumonias, an aggressive rather than conservative approach to diagnosis and therapy should be taken, as these infections often respond suboptimally to the usual therapies in the setting of severe immunosuppression. Early intervention is required for control or for eradication.

Late Post-Transplant Phase (Day >+100). In general, patients who reach this point are at less risk of serious infection. However, all patients remain immunosuppressed to some degree, and chronic GVHD patients especially have specific antibody production and T-cell abnormalities. Therefore, they remain at risk for infectious complications, chiefly with bacterial and viral organisms.

In the setting of chronic GVHD, bacterial infections (either local or disseminated), especially with encapsulated organisms such as *Streptococcus pneumoniae* and *Hemophilus influenzae*, are common. When these occur, prophylactic oral antibiotics (e.g., co-trimoxazole or penicillin) have been found effective. Conversely, immunization is usually not useful primarily due to poor antibody response. Viral infections are also common, and the infective interstitial pneumonitis due to cytomegalovirus that develops during this time is almost always seen in the setting of chronic GVHD. A more frequent complication is herpes zoster infections. These infections are seen frequently in patients without, but more frequently in those patients with, chronic GVHD. Although these infections usually remain localized, systemic acyclovir (500 mg/m^2 intravenously every 8 hours) is indicated for all cases of zoster with multi-dermatome or disseminated disease, and it may be useful for other patients as well. Rarely, Epstein-Barr virus infections may be associated with B-cell lymphoproliferative disease. Although no therapy has been proved effective, acyclovir and perhaps interferon may be useful.

The development of the acquired immunodeficiency disease syndrome (AIDS) may well be a problem of increasing importance in marrow transplantation, presumably due to transmission by blood products. Patients and donors should be screened for the human immunodeficiency virus (HIV) before transplantation, and patients should be checked again several months following transplantation. Infection with HIV should also be considered when patients have unexplained opportunistic infections later in their treatment courses than would otherwise be expected.

Donors

The infective history of the marrow donor must not be overlooked. While most donors are healthy, CMV, malaria, hepatitis B and human immunodeficiency virus reportedly have been transmitted in some cases. These infections may complicate or even contraindicate marrow transplantation.

Summary

An extremely wide variety of common and uncommon bacterial, fungal, viral and protozoal organisms produce infection after marrow transplantation. Such infections are a major complication of bone marrow transplantation, and are relatively predictable, considering the generalized immunosuppression and the sequential nature of immunologic recovery. To reduce infectious mortality, an aggressive approach to diagnosis as well as to therapy is recommended.

Many of the most serious infections are found in patients with severe GVHD. Therefore, while specific anti-infective measures may be developed for better prophylaxis and therapy, control of GVHD would greatly decrease the morbidity and mortality associated with infection.

The development of improved antimicrobial agents, especially those active against fungal and viral organisms, would also be most helpful. Likewise, the use of recombinant growth factors to shorten the period of immunosuppression, which will undoubtedly be explored within the next few years, potentially holds great promise.

References

Atkinson K, Biggs JC, Ting A, et al. (1983) Cyclosporin A is associated with faster engraftment and less mucositis than methotrexate after allogeneic bone marrow transplantation. Br J Haematol 53(2): 265

Bodey GP (1986) Fungal infection and fever of unknown origin in neutropenic patients. Am J Med 80 (Suppl 5C): 112

Bowden RA, Meyers JD (1985) Infectious complications following marrow transplantation. Plasma Ther Transfus Technol 6: 285

Bowden RA, Sayers M, Flournoy N, et al. (1986) Cytomegalovirus immune globulin and seronegative blood products to prevent primary cytomegalovirus infection after marrow transplantation. N Engl J Med 314: 1006

Karp JE, Dick JD, Angelopulos C, et al. (1986) Empiric use of vancomycin during prolonged treatment-induced granulocytopenia: Randomized, double-blind, placebo-controlled clinical trial in patients with acute leukemia. Am J Med 81: 237

Lum LG (1987) The kinetics of immune reconstitution after human marrow transplantation. Blood 69: 369

Meyers JD, Flournoy N, Thomas ED (1986) Risk factors for cytomegalovirus infection after human marrow transplantation. J Infect Dis 153: 478

Noel DR, Witherspoon RP, Storb R, et al. (1978) Does graft-versus-host disease influence the tempo of immunologic recovery after allogeneic human marrow transplantation? An observation on 56 long-term survivors. Blood 51: 1087

Peterson FB, Clift RA, Hickman RO, et al. (1986) Hickman catheter complications in marrow transplant recipients. J Parenteral and Enteral Nutrition 10: 58

Pizzo PA, Hathorn JW, Hiemenz J, et al. (1986) A randomized trial comparing ceftazidime alone with combination antibiotic therapy in cancer patients with fever and neutropenia. N Engl J Med 315: 552

Saral R (1985) Viral infections in bone marrow transplantation recipients. Plasma Ther Transfus Technol 6: 275

Shearer WT, Ritz J, Finegold MJ, et al. (1985) Epstein-Barr virus-associated B-cell proliferations of diverse clonal origins after bone marrow transplantation in a 12-year-old patient with severe combined immunodeficiency. N Engl J Med 312: 1151

Shepp DH, Dandliker PS, de Miranda P, et al. (1985) Activity of 9-[2-Hydroxy-1-(hydroxymethyl)ethoxymethyl]guanine in the treatment of cytomegalovirus pneumonia. Ann Int Med 103: 368

Storb R, Doney KC, Thomas ED, et al. (1982) Marrow transplantation with or without donor buffy coat cells for 65 transfused aplastic anemia patients. Blood 59: 236

Storb R, Thomas ED, Buckner CD, et al. (1980) Marrow transplantation in thirty "untransfused" patients with severe aplastic anemia. Ann Int Med 92: 30

Winston DJ, Ho WG, Lin C-H, et al. (1987) Intravenous immune globulin for prevention of cytomegalovirus infection and interstitial pneumonia after bone marrow transplantation. Ann Int Med 106: 12

Young LS (1984) An overview of infection in bone marrow transplant recipients. Clin Haematol 13: 661

5. Interstitial Pneumonitis

Definition

Interstitial pneumonitis is usually defined as a nonbacterial, nonfungal pneumonitis. The disease process involves mostly the pulmonary interstitium in the form of mononuclear cell infiltration and fluid accumulation with a relative sparing of air spaces. Because of this, there is only little productive cough, and it may be difficult to establish the diagnosis on the basis of sputum cultures or bronchoalveolar lavage. Radiographically, the process can be localized or diffuse with a prominent interstitial pattern. Although the clinical picture with shortness of breath, hypoxemia, and radiographic findings is rather typical, a definitive diagnosis often requires an open lung biopsy.

Etiology

Several etiological factors for the development of interstitial pneumonitis have been recognized (Table 18). The most important cause at the present time is cytomegalovirus which accounts for almost half the cases of interstitial pneumonitis observed after marrow transplantation. In another large fraction of

Table 18. Etiology of Interstitial Pneumonitis

1. Infections		
	Viruses	– Cytomegalovirus (CMV)
		– Herpes simplex virus (HSV)
		– Varicella-zoster virus (VZV)
		– Adenovirus
		– Respiratory syncytial virus
		– Measles virus
	Pneumocystis carinii	
	Legionella	
	Chlamydia trachomatis	
2. Irradiation		
3. Chemical Causes		
	– Cyclophosphamide	
	– Busulfan	
	– Methotrexate	
4. Idiopathic		

patients no infectious agent can be identified and these cases are listed under the heading "idiopathic" interstitial pneumonitis. It is thought, however, that idiopathic pneumonitis is at least in part related to irradiation, and possibly to chemotherapy. All other etiologies are less frequent. In earlier studies Pneumocystis carinii was found in as many as 10–15% of cases. However, since initiation of trimethoprim/sulfamethoxazole prophylaxis, the incidence has declined substantially. All other causes listed are quite infrequent.

Risk Factors and Epidemiology

Several risk factors have been identified (Table 19). Interstitial pneumonitis can occur as early as one week and as late as two years after transplantation. However, the peak incidence is at approximately 8–10 weeks. Idiopathic interstitial pneumonitis tends to occur somewhat earlier than CMV related pneumonitis. As one might expect, recognized risk factors differ for cases of interstitial pneumonitis tied to different etiologies.

Patients given an allogeneic transplant have a significantly higher probability of developing CMV pneumonitis than patients given a syngeneic or autologous transplant. In fact, in the first 100 patients given a syngeneic transplant in Seattle, no case of CMV pneumonitis was identified. In agreement with the concept that allogenecity contributes to the development of CMV pneumonitis is the observation that this entity increases in frequency with the severity of GVHD in the recipient. No such correlation has been recognized for idiopathic interstitial pneumonitis, which appears to occur with similar frequency in patients given allogeneic or syngeneic transplants, and in patients with and without acute GVHD.

Patients transplanted for the treatment of severe aplastic anemia have a lower incidence of interstitial pneumonitis than patients transplanted for lymphohemopoietic malignancies. Although it is conceivable that the underlying diagnosis itself represents a risk factor, it is clear that the conditioning used in preparation for transplantation is of importance. Until recently most patients with lymphohemopoietic malignancies were conditioned with regimens including the use

Table 19. Risk Factors for the Development of Interstitial Pneumonitis After Marrow Transplantation

- Allogeneic transplant
- Graft-vs-host disease
- Total body irradiation (TBI) for conditioning
- Higher exposure rate used for TBI
- Single dose TBI
- Prior radiotherapy to the chest
- Seropositivity for cytomegalovirus (CMV)
- Transfusion of CMV positive blood products
- Increasing patient age
- Methotrexate post-transplant
- Female donor sex
- Omission of trimethoprim/sulfamethoxazole prophylaxis

of TBI, most patients with non-malignant disorders such as severe aplastic anemia have been conditioned with chemotherapy only or, if TBI was used, generally at lower total doses than in patients with lymphohemopoietic malignancies. Subsequently, it was observed that the incidence of interstitial pneumonitis declined with the use of fractionated rather than single dose TBI. It was of note, however, that TBI dose fractionation had its impact mostly on idiopathic interstitial pneumonitis, and affected very little the incidence of CMV related pneumonitis. The beneficial effect of fractionated TBI on idiopathic interstitial pneumonitis was particularly prominent in patients who were given methotrexate rather than cyclosporine as GVHD prophylaxis. There is also evidence that patients with a diagnosis of Hodgkin's disease or non-Hodgkin's lymphoma, who previously received irradiation to the chest or the mediastinum have sa significantly higher probability of developing idiopathic interstitial pneumonitis than patients without prior radiotherapy. Furthermore, a recent analysis by the International Bone Marrow Transplantation Registry suggests that patients given TBI at an exposure rate of $\geq$ 5.7 cGy/min have a higher incidence of pneumonitis than patients irradiated at lower exposure rates. The second most significant risk factor for the development of CMV pneumonitis next to acute GVHD is the CMV immune status of the patient. The lowest incidence of CMV pneumonitis is observed in patients who have no evidence of prior exposure to CMV, and who are being transplanted from a similarly CMV negative donor. If the donor is positive for CMV, the risk of developing significant CMV infection even in a CMV negative recipient, increases substantially. If the patient himself is CMV positive, the risk increases further, and does not appear to be significantly affected by the donor CMV status. Consequently, the transfusion of CMV positive blood products also represents a risk factor for CMV pneumonitis, at least in patients who are CMV negative.

An additional risk factor is patient age. Although one component may be that CMV positivity is lower in young patients than in older patients, age by itself was found to be an independent factor in a recent analysis of the Seattle data.

Other risk factors that have been described such as female donor sex, the interval from diagnosis to transplant and the performance rating before transplantation are more controversial.

Of interest are recent findings reported by Sullivan and colleagues. These investigators found that patients who developed chronic GVHD and were not given treatment had an approximate 15% probability of developing late interstitial pneumonitis. If these patients received treatment for GVHD, the probability increased to approximately 30%. If, however, in addition to treatment for GVHD, infection prophylaxis in the form of trimethoprim/sulfamethoxazole was given, the probability of interstitial pneumonitis was only 8%.

Pathogenesis

As shown in Table 18 interstitial pneumonitis can have several etiologies. The presence of an infectious agent in the immunosuppressed patient will lead to an inflammatory reaction, presumably facilitated by a direct toxic effect of the conditioning regimen on pulmonary tissue. This inflammatory reaction involves mononuclear cell infiltration and fluid accumulation and leads to thickening of the interstitium. As a consequence, the diffusing distance for oxygen from the air space (alveoli) to the capillaries in the interstitium increases and arterial oxygen concentration in the blood decreases. The patient senses hypoxemia and feels short of breath. Early in the course, only partial arterial oxygen pressure will fall and as a consequence of increased respiratory effort, pCO_2 may be lower than normal. There may be a mild degree of respiratory alkalosis. As the patient tires, there may be a slowly increasing retention of CO_2 in addition to hypoxemia. Along with a hypoxemic metabolism this will result in a combined metabolic/respiratory acidosis. As the patient is being treated by increased oxygen intake (FiO_2) initially by mask, and subsequently often via endotracheal intubation, there may be secondary damage to the alveolar lining due to prolonged high oxygen exposure. The end result is a wet, heavy, and stiff lung incapable of performing its functions.

Clinical and Laboratory Features

The interstitial process leads to hypoxemia with air hunger and shortness of breath. Auscultation of the lung may be completely unrevealing, and in fact the lungs may be suspiciously silent. There may be some nonspecific crackling sounds. A chest radiograph, however, as described above, shows interstitial markings which can be localized or, more frequently, diffuse. These markings can involve the bases of the lungs, the perihilar areas, or can lead to a complete "white out" of both lung fields (Fig. 6a, b and 7). Usually there will be fever but an occasional patient may be afebrile, which is not surprising since many patients are on immunosuppressive therapy including steroids. Although the clinical picture of interstitial pneumonitis is rather typical, a conclusion as to its etiology is often not possible.

Sputum is hardly ever available for examination. Brochoalveolar lavages and transbrochial biopsies are often inadequate to establish a diagnosis. The most reliable diagnostic procedure is open lung biopsy. Although there may be concern about hemorrhage during and following the procedure, usually adequate platelet support can be provided to prevent major hemorrhages. Histological examination will reveal mononuclear cell infiltrates and fluid exudation into the interstitial space. There may be hemorrhage as well. In the case of CMV infection, characteristic intranuclear or cytoplasmatic inclusion bodies can be found (Fig. 6a, b). In addition, virus may grow in culture. Concurrently, there may be an increase in the antibody titer against CMV as determined by complement fixation techniques or enzyme linked immunosorption assay. More recently monoclonal antibodies have become available that recognize certain protein structures of the virus which can be directly visualized by fluorescence techniques. As a research tool in situ hybridization with DNA probes complementary to certain CMV sequences can be utilized. Concurrently with the development of pneumonitis, CMV may be present in the intestinal mucosa, liver or blood, or may be excreted in the urine.

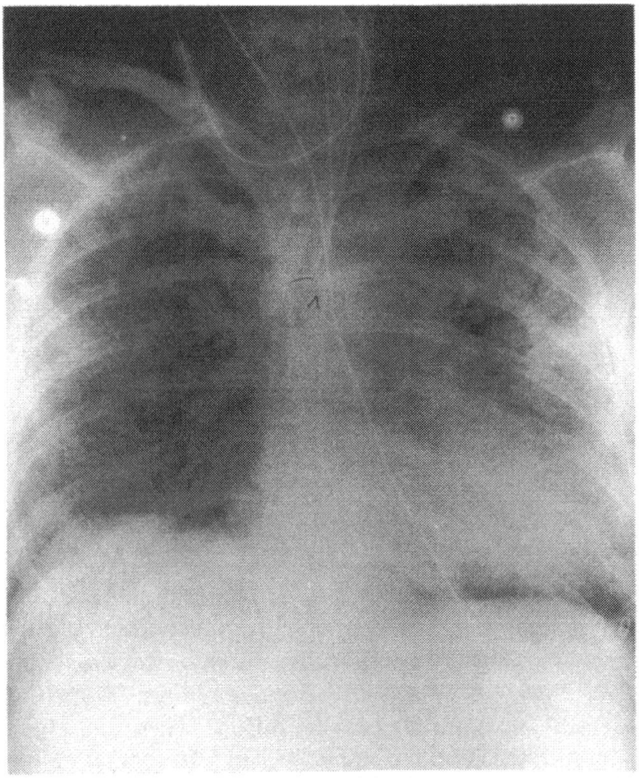

a

Fig. 6a, b. Interstitial pneumonitis. Diffuse interstitial markings in both lung fields with a "white out" appearance in the left lower lobe (a). Tissue obtained at open lung biopsy reveals giant cells with cytoplasmatic and nuclear viral inclusion bodies characteristic of cytomegalovirus (b)

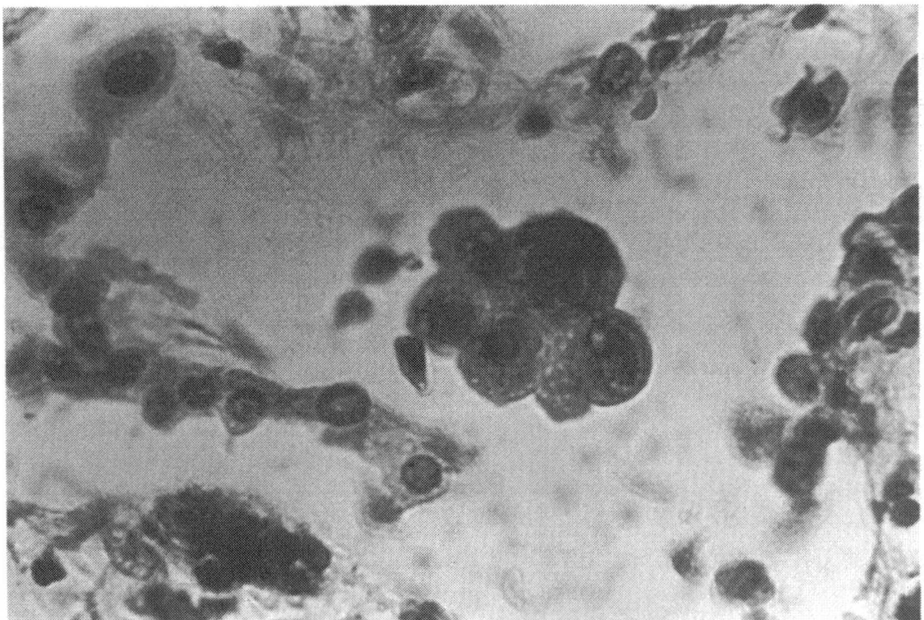

b

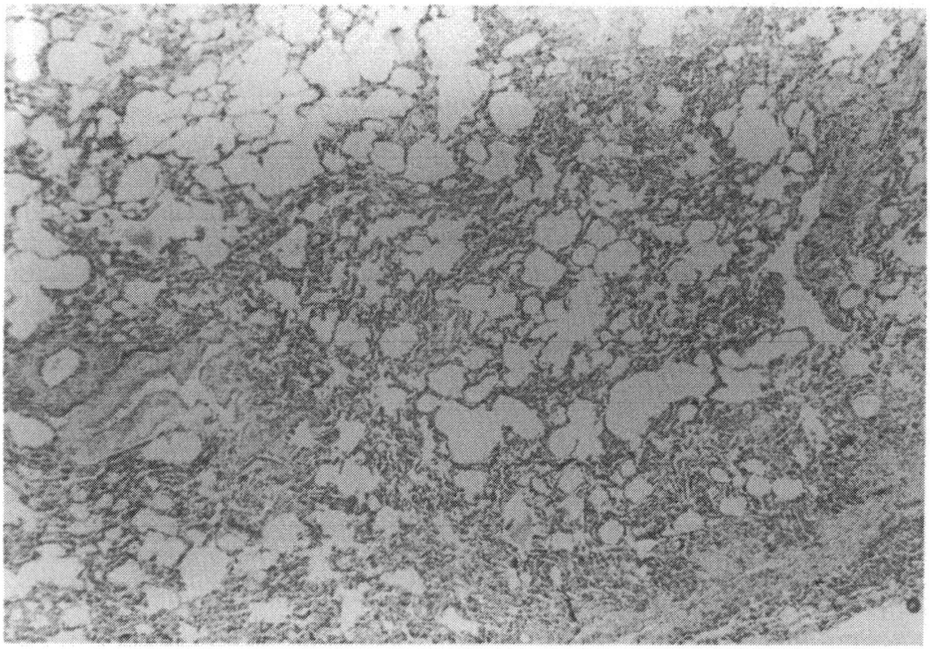

Fig. 7. Idiopathic interstitial pneumonitis showing thickened alveolar septa with edema and round cell infiltrates. No organisms identified

Pneumocystis carinii pneumonitis is diagnosed when cysts of the organism are demonstrated in pulmonary tissue sections using stains such as silver methenamine or toluidine blue. In an occasional patient Pneumocystis can also be diagnosed from bronchial washings.

Herpes simplex virus, varicella zoster virus and adenovirus also cause inclusion bodies in cells of lung tissue. Some of them grow well in cultures causing characteristic cytopathic effects. Similar to the diagnosis of CMV pneumonitis, fluorescein labeled monoclonal antibodies specific for these viruses are now available for diagnostic purposes. Interstitial pneumonitis due to herpes virus frequently occurs in the setting of disseminated infection also involving the skin.

If complete examination of the tissue obtained at biopsy fails to reveal any organism, although the histological appearance is typical, usually the diagnosis of idiopathic interstitial pneumonitis is made (Fig. 7). It is thought that irradiation and chemical agents as listed in Table 18 contribute to the development of this entity.

Differential Diagnosis

A patient presenting with shortness of breath, fever, and diffuse interstitial changes on chest radiograph is always suspected of having interstitial pneumonitis until proven otherwise. Fluid overload has to be excluded as an etiology, particularly if the picture develops early after transplantation, and in a setting of veno-occlusive disease of the liver or generalized capillary leak syndrome associated with a significant increase in body weight. An aggressive trial with diuretics provides a rapid answer since there will be no improvement in the case of interstitial pneumonitis. Conceivably, a diffuse fungal pneumonia could resemble interstitial pneumonitis. Such a diagnosis is suspected when fungus, particularly Candida species, is grown from various culture sites including the sputum, but it may be necessary to obtain lung tissue to confirm the diagnosis. An acute respiratory distress syndrome may remotely resemble interstitial pneumonitis. The clinical picture with associated septicemia will be helpful. Organisms such as Mycobacteria or Chlamydia may rarely cause pneumonitis, and the diagnosis will depend upon documentation of the organisms in tissue or the results of cultures.

Treatment and Prognosis

Approximately 40% of all cases of interstitial pneumonitis are related to CMV. Mortality with CMV pneumonitis has been reported to be 85–90%. Agents such as vidarabine, interferon, and acyclovir have been used for treatment but have not significantly altered the disease course. The median survival was approximately 3 weeks after diagnosis. Recent investigational studies suggest that the use of high dose immunoglobulin containing anti-CMV activity or even a combination of immunoglobulin and acyclovir may arrest the disease in a proportion of patients and reduce mortality.

Pneumocystis carinii pneumonitis is usually treated with trimethoprim-sulfamethoxazole, which allows recovery in approximately 80–90% of patients.

The rare cases of herpes simplex virus or varicella-zoster virus pneumonitis are treated most effectively with acyclovir.

No treatment is available for adenovirus.

Mortality with idiopathic interstitial pneumonitis is in the range of 50–60%. Many investigators have used high dose corticosteroids, and feel this is effective although no controlled study has been performed.

Prevention

Risk factors for the development of interstitial pneumonitis have been discussed above. Since CMV related interstitial pneumonitis is most frequent, many researchers have focused on this entity. Several studies have shown that patients transplanted from CMV positive donors, and in addition given granulocyte transfusions, are at the highest risk of developing CMV pneumonitis. The omission of granulocyte transfusions clearly reduced the incidence of CMV excretion, and subsequent symptomatic disease in these patients. A recent analysis of 540 patients studied in Seattle revealed the following: patients who were CMV negative at the time of transplantation and who were transplanted from a CMV negative donor had a probability of approximately 20% of subsequently excreting CMV; if the donor was CMV positive, the probability increased to 40%. If the patient was CMV positive at the time of transplantation, the donor CMV status did not appear to affect the outcome, and approximately 60% of patients excreted CMV. It is thought that in those instances where both donor and recipient were CMV negative, CMV infection was due to the transfusion of CMV positive blood products. Consequently, all CMV negative patients should be given CMV negative blood products; in CMV positive patients the administration of CMV positive blood products does not appear to further increase the pre-existing substantial risk of developing CMV infection. Overall the risk of developing CMV interstitial pneumonitis in CMV positive patients was twice as high as in CMV negative patients. Several recent studies have examined the usefulness of longterm administration of gamma globulin preparations with high titers of antibody to CMV. A consensus appears to be developing that this approach is beneficial. Although in some studies the rate of CMV infection was not altered, CMV disease was decreased; in other studies both infection and disease incidence were lower in the treatment group. Investigations are underway to develop a CMV vaccine but this approach is not clinically available yet.

Pneumocystis carinii pneumonitis can be prevented almost completely by the prophylactic administration of trimethoprim-sulfamethoxazole beginning before transplantation and given for two days a week after transplantation for approximately 6 months in patients without GVHD; longer for patients with GVHD (see below).

The incidence of idiopathic interstitial pneumonitis has decreased with the use of fractionated rather than single dose TBI. The beneficial effect of fractionation appears to be particularly prominent in patients given methotrexate for GVHD prophylaxis but was also noticeable in patients given cyclosporine. Overall the incidence of idiopathic interstitial pneumonitis has decreased from approximately 13% with single dose TBI to 5% with fractionated TBI.

The development of acute GVHD increases the risk of CMV pneumonitis 2–3 times as compared to patients without GVHD. Consequently, every attempt must be made to reduce or prevent the development of GVHD. The use of a combination of methotrexate and cyclosporine or T-cell depletion have proven useful for GVHD prevention but their beneficial effect in regards to interstitial pneumonitis remains to be proven. If GVHD develops and treatment is necessary, the use of antithymocyte globulin further increases the risk of CMV pneumonitis, and it might be advisable to use other agents such as steroids for treatment.

While the risk of interstitial pneumonitis in patients without chronic GVHD is limited to the first two to four months after transplantation, patients who develop extensive chronic GVHD may be at risk for several years following transplantation. In a recent report Sullivan et al. described late interstitial pneumonitis in 28 of 198 patients. It was idiopathic in 23%, due to CMV in 19%, due to pneumocystis in 19%, and varicella zoster in 10%. Half of the patients died. These investigators showed that the probability of developing late interstitial pneumonitis was approximately 30% in patients who were not given antibiotic prophylaxis, but was only 8% in patients who received prophylactic trimethoprim/sulfamethoxazole. The beneficial effect of this drug was mostly although not exclusively due to prevention of pneumocystis carinii pneumonitis.

These data clearly indicate that the prevention of both acute and chronic GVHD is desirable in order to prevent interstitial pneumonitis. Whether prolonged prophylactic administration of immunoglobulin preparations as currently being investigated will prevent interstitial pneumonitis remains to be determined. Also, it is not clear whether obstructive and restrictive pulmonary abnormalities that have been observed late after marrow transplantation are related to an interstitial pneumonitis process that has gone unrecognized.

References

Barrett A, Depledge MH, Powles RL (1983) Interstitial pneumonitis following bone marrow transplantation after low dose rate total body irradiation. Int J Radiation Oncology Biol Phys 9: 1029

Condie R O'Reilly RJ (1984) Prevention of cytomegalovirus infection by prophylaxis with an intravenous, hyperimmune, native, unmodified cytomegalovirus globulin: Randomized trial in bone marrow transplant recipients. Am J Med 76: 134

Emanuel D, Peppard J, Stover D, Gold J, Armstrong D, Hammerling U (1986) Rapid immunodiagnosis of cytomegalovirus pneumonia by bronchoalveolar lavage using human and muring monoclonal antibodies. Ann Int Med 104: 476

Griffiths PD, Stirk PR, Blacklock HA, Milburn HJ, du Bois RM, Prentice HG (1987) Rapid diagnosis and treatment of cytomegalovirus pneumonitis. Progress in Bone Marrow Transplantation RP Gale and R Champlin (eds) Alan R Liss, Inc., New York pp. 583

Kubanek B, Ernst P, Ostendorf P, Schafer U, Wolf H (1985) Preliminary data of a controlled trial of intravenous hyperimmune globulin in the prevention of cytomegalovirus infection in bone marrow transplant recipients. Transplant Proc 17: 468

Lonnqvist B, Ringden O, Wahren B, Gahrton G, Lundgren G (1984) Cytomegalovirus infection associated with and preceding chronic graft-versus-host disease. Transplantation 38: 465

Meyers JD, Flournoy N, Thomas ED (1986) Risk factors for cytomegalovirus infection after human marrow transplantation. J Infect Dis 153: 478

Meyers JD, Shepp DH, Bowden RA, Reed EC (1987) Viral infections in marrow transplant recipients. Progress in Bone Marrow Transplantation RP Gale and R Champlin (eds) Alan R Liss, Inc., New York, pp 545

Miller WM, Flynn P, McCullough J, Balfour HH, Goldman A, Haake, R, McGlave P, Ramsay N, Kersey J (1986) Cytomegalovirus infection after bone marrow transplantation: an association with acute graft-v-host disease. Blood 67: 1162

Shields AF, Hackman RC, Fife KH, Corey L, Meyers JD (1985) Adenovirus infections in patients undergoing bone-marrow transplantation. New Eng J Med 312: 529

Teshima, H, Masaoka T, Inoue T, Kato S, Naito K, Mori T, Kanamaru A, Saito Y, Ohira M, Moryama Y, Kodera Y, Harada M, Baba M, Nakade Y, Tasaka H, Yoshikawa S (1986) Interstitial pneumonitis in allogeneic bone marrow transplantation: a report from the Japanese BMT study group. Bone Marrow Transplantation 1: 179

Torres JL, Bross DS, Lam WC, Wharam MD, Santos GW, Order SE (1982) Risk factors in interstitial pneumonitis following allogeneic bone marrow transplantation. Int J Radiation Oncology Biol Phys 8: 1301

Weiner RS, Bortin MM, Gale RP, Gluckman E, Kay HEM, Kolb HJ, Hartz AJ, Rimm AA (1986) Interstitial pneumonitis after bone marrow transplantation. Ann Int Med 104: 168

Winston DJ, Ho WG, Gale RP, Champlin RE (1987) Treatment and prevention of interstitial pneumonia after bone marrow transplantation. Progress in Bone Marrow Transplantation RP Gale and R Champlin (eds) Alan R Liss, Inc., New York, pp 525

Zaia J A and Churchill M A (1987) The biology of human cytomegalovirus infection after marrow transplation. Progress in Bone Marrow Transplantation. Progress in Bone Marrow Transplantation R. P. Gale and R. Champlin (eds) Alan R. Liss, Inc., New York pp 563

6. Hepatic Dysfunction

Jaundice frequently occurs after marrow transplantation. Time course, treatment and prognosis are different for each clinical entity and the following diseases have to be distinguished:
- Veno-occlusive disease (VOD)
- Acute GVHD
- Chronic GVHD
- Infection
- Drug Injury
- Parenteral Nutrition
- Recurrent Tumor

Veno-Occlusive Disease (VOD)

VOD is generally believed to be a consequence of toxic injury to the liver resulting from high dose chemoradiotherapy used to condition the patient. In certain disease categories, and age groups, it is the most common liver disease in the first month posttransplant.

VOD is seldom seen in patients with aplastic anemia prepared with cyclophosphamide alone. In contrast, about 20–30% of patients with malignancy prepared with a combination of chemotherapy and total body irradiation develop VOD. The incidence in patients undergoing autologous transplantation is only 5%. For unknown reasons, VOD appears to occur less often in patients after syngeneic transplantation, although the doses of chemoradiotherapy are similar to those used for allogeneic transplantation.

Pathogenesis

Active metabolites of antineoplastic agents may be concentrated in the pericentral zone of the liver sinusoids, reaching toxic concentrations. The sinusoidal blood flow can then be obstructed by injured and necrotic hepatocytes, and, in addition, sinusoidal pores may be blocked by cellular debris and exfoliated hepatocytes. This can cause a shift of fluid containing sodium and albumin from the intravascular to the extravascular space ("third space"). Since renal blood flow decreases, the kidneys react by activating the renin-angiotensin mechanism resulting in sodium retention. The clinical picture ultimately consists of *hepatomegaly, abdominal pain, peripheral fluid accumulation, ascites,* and *impaired liver function with icterus.* In severe cases with prolonged liver dysfunction, renal insufficiency may develop secondary to prerenal failure and toxic tubular damage.

In cyclosporine treated patients, an additional pathogenetic mechanism is thought to occur. Cyclosporine reduces prostacyclin release from endothelial cells, which in turn may cause coagulation abnormalities and facilitate capillary thrombosis. Cyclosporine treated patients also have elevated levels of coagulation factor VIII, and fibrinogen as well as increased aggregation of platelets. Therefore, cyclosporine-induced coagulation abnormalities may be superimposed on chemotherapy/radiation related hepatic damage and contribute to the development of VOD.

Histopathology

Early changes include centrilobular hemorrhage, subendothelial edema, and intimal proliferation. Intermediate changes are characterized by the occlusion of the venular lumen by collagen fibers (subendothelial), and atrophy of pericentral hepatocytes. Late changes may show recanalization of venules, centrilobular cholestasis, and an overall abnormal lobular architecture.

Risk Factors

- presence of active hepatocellular disease at the time of transplantation (increases the risk of VOD three to four times)
- history of hepatitis
- older patient age
- intensity of conventional chemotherapy prior to transplantation
- intensity and type of preparative regimen
- diagnosis (more frequent with CML).

There is no correlation, however, between any of these risk factors and the severity of VOD. In terms of age, VOD is more often seen in recipients over the age of 15. The incidence of VOD is also higher in patients prepared with total body irradiation in combination with chemotherapy. Radiation seems to be an important cause of VOD, since VOD was not observed in 200 patients transplanted for aplastic anemia conditioned only with cyclophosphamide. Also, VOD is seen more often when high dose cytosine-arabinoside is added to a regimen consisting of cyclophosphamide and total body irradiation. Moreover, the use of more than two alkylating agents predisposes to the development of VOD. Thus, VOD is more often seen in patients who are receiving a second transplant and are, for example, prepared with a combination of busulfan and cyclophosphamide (both alkylating agents). The administration of cyclosporine during the preparative period together with high dose chemoradiotherapy is also associated with an increase in the incidence of VOD as shown in patients transplanted for aplastic anemia. Cyclosporine and cyclophosphamide are hepatotoxic when given individually. Cyclosporine can cause centrilobular necrosis, and cylophosphamide has been reported to depress hepatic microsomal enzymes. Other drugs, such as dacarbazine, BCNU, 6-thioguanine and mitomycin C, have all been related to VOD. Despite an early report suggesting that VOD could be a manifestation of GVHD, no such correlation has been found in subsequent investigations in larger numbers of patients. Methotrexate is generally not thought to cause hepatic problems in this setting.

In patients with unexplained elevated liver function tests prior to marrow transplantation, a liver biopsy should be obtained. If it shows active hepatitis, it is recommended that marrow transplantation be postponed until liver function tests have returned to normal. A liver biopsy may also clarify whether elevated liver function tests are secondary to liver involvement by leukemia or lymphoma, in which case the risk of VOD is not increased and marrow transplantation should not be delayed.

Diagnosis

Signs and symptoms of VOD usually develop within three weeks of transplantation. *Weight gain* due to fluid retention and *jaundice* are often noticed first, followed by *hepatomegaly* and *abdominal pain* usually in the right upper quadrant. The diagnosis of VOD is likely if at least two of these features are present before day 30 posttransplant. With more severe VOD, ascites and hepatic encephalopathy may also develop. Usually levels of serum transaminases and alkaline phosphatase are only mildly or moderately elevated, and may rise later than the bilirubin.

Clinical Course

VOD can present as a mild illness with complete recovery or as rapidly progressive hepatic failure with encephalopathy and ensuing death. Data from Seattle indicate that VOD resolves in the majority of patients (55%) but contributes to death in about 30% of those who develop clinically manifest VOD. When hepatic function is significantly impaired with high bilirubin and low serum albumin, a picture reminiscent of hepatorenal syndrome with renal failure may develop. Patients with severe VOD tend to have higher peak values for bilirubin and aspartate aminotransferase as well as a more significant weight gain than patients with a mild form of VOD. Persistent jaundice along with ascites is considered a poor prognostic sign.

With an uncomplicated course, serum bilirubin and enzyme abnormalities may return to normal within 3–4 weeks. However, since acute GVHD may develop at about the same time, a delayed resolution of signs from previously diagnosed VOD can be observed. Since the therapeutic management for VOD and GVHD differs, a correct tissue diagnosis, whenever obtainable, is helpful.

Interestingly, patients with mild VOD do not have markedly abnormal coagulation parameters, and replacement therapy in the form of plasma cryoprecipitate, fresh plasma, and/or coagulation factor concentrates is rarely indicated.

Differential Diagnosis

Jaundice, hepatomegaly, and ascites may be nonspecific findings (Table 20). However, their development early after transplantation (e.g. weight gain or increasing bilirubin on day 3 or 4 post transplant) is highly suggestive of VOD, although congestive heart failure, viral hepatitis and intra-abdominal sepsis must be excluded. Liver damage due to cyclosporine alone or in combination with methotrexate may also cause icterus, but, in these cases the total bilirubin usually does not exceed 5 mg% (85 μmol/l). Furthermore, jaundice together with ascites or significant weight gain (or both) are usually not seen in drug-induced hepatic damage. Acute GVHD of the liver seldom manifests before the third week after transplant, and usually does not present with ascites. In an occasional patient, however, symptoms of VOD may develop later and it might be impossible to establish an accurate diagnosis without liver histology.

Table 20. Differential Diagnosis of Jaundice Early after Transplantation

	Diagnosis			
	VOD	Acute GVHD	Hepatitis	Cyclosporine Toxicity
Onset (days post BMT)	0–25	>15	0–100	>0
Transaminases	0–↑	↑↑	↑↑↑	0
Alkaline Phosphatase	↑↑	↑	↑↑	0–↑
Weight gain	+++	–	–	–
Liver failure	possible	rare	possible	no

Diagnostic Procedures

- Ultrasound and computed tomography may show a congested liver and can usually exclude the presence of an abscess or infiltrative processes.
- A liver biopsy can be useful to distinguish VOD, acute GVHD and infection of the liver as well as obstruction of hepatic veins by fungus. Since patients are generally severely thrombocytopenic early after transplantation, a liver biopsy is associated with an increased risk of hemorrhage. Attempts must be made to raise the platelet count to 50–60 $\times$ 10^9/L and maintain it at that level for $\simeq$ 24–36 hours after the procedure. There is also an increased risk of bleeding due to congested veins, and an associated coagulopathy.

Treatment

Therapeutic options are limited to symptomatic measures. A negative sodium balance should be achieved by restriction of sodium intake. Parenteral nutrition solutions are concentrated to reduce total volume and free water but prevent the development of a catabolic state. Also, carefully balanced electrolyte solutions must be used. Concentrated dextrose solution is not contraindicated. Lipid emulsions are controversial. However, as much as 50% of total calories can be supplied in the form of lipids. Intravenous volume and renal perfusion must be maintained. Albumin (25 g iv two to four times daily), despite its short intravascular half life, may be helpful in maintaining the serum albumin levels and the respective osmotic pressures.

Hematocrit should be maintained at a level of ≥ 0.30 (hemoglobin at ≥ 100 g/l) with transfusion of packed red blood cells, since erythrocytes contribute to the total osmotic load, and provide sufficient oxygen to hepatocytes.

Spironolactone is recommended if the creatinine is < 1.2 mg/dl (< 106 µmol/l) and the patient can swallow the tablets. Alternatively, the use of furosemide in small doses (10–20 mg iv) in conjunction with transfusions may help maintain renal perfusion. Furosemide must be used cautiously, particularly in patients on cyclosporine in whom renal function is already impaired. Its effect on sodium balance is also unpredictable. In severe VOD, hemofiltration has been used to remove volume and sodium, but generally with little success. The use of low-dose dopamine (2 µg/kg/min) to increase renal blood flow is still controversial, but is used by many investigators.

Hepatic encephalopathy should be treated with oral protein restriction and possibly lactulose (side effect: diarrhea). Although studies are not yet conclusive, the infusion of high-branched chain amino acid solutions (Hepatamine) is preferred. Drugs which are predominantly metabolized by the liver, such as cyclosporine and methotrexate, need dose adjustment or must be omitted. It is also important to use sedatives and analgetics cautiously. Due to impaired hepatic metabolism, drugs and their metabolites can accumulate, and cause an altered level of consciousness in these patients. Meperidine (Demerol®), morphine and various benzodiazepines in particular can result in a picture which may mimic hepatic encephalopathy.

Acute GVHD (see also IV.2)

Pathogenesis

Experimental data suggest that lymphohemopoetic cells are the primary target of the immunologic attack in GVHD. The mechanisms of hepatocyte necrosis are unknown, but may be explained by an "innocent bystander" reaction.

Histopathology

Early changes may show mild nonspecific lobular hepatitis and infiltration of mononuclear cells and eosinophils in the portal triads. Intermediate changes include cholestasis, an infiltration of portal zones by lymphocytes, and destruction of small bile ducts by abnormal interlobular proliferation. Late changes can show profound cholestasis, degeneration of peripheral hepatocytes, and reduction in the number of bile ducts by abnormal interlobular proliferation.

Diagnosis

In the majority of patients skin and intestinal involvement by acute GVHD is present concurrently, and may suggest the diagnosis of acute GVHD of the liver (see IV.2). Signs of severe liver function impairment such as acute liver failure with ascites and encephalopathy, and reduced synthesis of coagulation factors are uncommon. Serum alkaline phosphatase may steadily increase with or without a parallel rise in bilirubin, and transaminases are usually moderately elevated. In an occasional patient, it might be necessary to obtain a liver biopsy, especially when additional signs of GVHD (skin/gut) are not present, and a differential diagnosis of VOD, hepatitis or drug-induced liver damage cannot be made with certainty.

Clinical Course

In mild cases an elevation of serum alkaline phosphatase without icterus may be the only sign. In more severe cases, a striking elevation of serum bilirubin can occur. Complications of hepatic failure such as encephalopathy, ascites and hepatorenal syndrome are uncommon, and death associated with acute liver GVHD in these patients is the exception. However, since severe GVHD in general, and its immunosuppressive treatment in particular, aggravate immunodeficiency after BMT, overwhelming infections are the most frequent cause of death in these patients.

Treatment

Modalities of treatment of acute GVHD are described above (IV 2). Even with treatment, acute GVHD of the liver may take weeks to months to resolve completely.

Chronic GVHD (see also V.2)

About 90% of all patients with chronic GVHD will show some degree of hepatic involvement, either as part of an extensive GVHD process or as a more limited disease involving only skin and liver. About 30–40% of long term survivors after allogeneic marrow grafting may have signs of chronic GVHD of the liver.

Pathogenesis

The main targets of chronic GVHD of the liver are the small interlobular bile ducts. However, the pathogenesis of their destruction and how this is immunologically mediated is largely hypothetical. Since bile duct cells express Class II histocompatibility (HLA-DR, DP, DQ) antigens, cytotoxic action of donor lymphocytes against these cells is likely to be involved.

Histopathology

Histologic examination may show signs of active or persistent chronic hepatitis with portal inflammation and fibrosis, degeneration of bile ducts, and dense plasmacytic infiltrates in the portal area.

Diagnosis

In the majority of cases, other organs are also affected by chronic GVHD. Serum alkaline phosphatase is usually elevated to 5–10 times normal. If the liver appears to be the only organ involved, a biopsy may be necessary to exclude other causes of hepatic dysfunction. In some patients a persistently elevated alkaline phosphatase may represent residual damage to the intrahepatic biliary tree rather than active chronic GVHD.

Clinical Course

The intensity of jaundice can fluctuate in parallel with the activity of chronic GVHD in other organ systems. Portal hypertension, hepatic failure and cirrhosis as a consequence of chronic GVHD are rare but have been observed. In two reported cases with chronic GVHD who developed hepatic failure, one showed cirrhosis and the other had an intact lobular architecture but absence of small bile ducts.

With treatment, an elevated alkaline phosphatase will usually decline within 3–4 weeks unless there is persistent damage to the biliary system. A flare-up of chronic GVHD may be heralded by increasing alkaline phosphatase levels. Prolonged treatment for 9 months or more may be necessary. About half of the patients will remain free of chronic GVHD after immunosuppression is stopped. In some patients chronic GVHD of the liver may develop de novo after day 100 post marrow transplantation. The primary physician should contact a transplant center to obtain information as to further management of the patient.

Treatment

Both limited (confined to the liver) and extensive chronic GVHD require treatment. Cyclosporine either alone or in combination with steroids has been proven to be effective (for details see IV 2).

Infections of the Liver

Based on an analysis of biopsy and autopsy material, the most common infections of the liver in marrow transplant recipients are of viral etiology. Several viruses can cause hepatitis: non-A – non-B, hepatitis B virus, cytomegalovirus (CMV), and less often, adenovirus, varicella zoster (VZV) and herpes simplex (HSV).

Viral Infections

Non A – non B Hepatitis and Hepatitis B

Many patients with aplastic anemia and leukemia are exposed to non-A – non-B hepatitis virus (δ-agent) because of their extensive transfusion requirements. In over half the patients with acute leukemia, a smoldering type of chronic hepatitis develops. Histological studies demonstrate nonspecific lobular hepatitis or chronic active hepatitis is presumably transfusion acquired either before or after transplantaton. Since blood products are now screened for hepatitis B virus, the likelihood of acquiring hepatitis B infection today is not very high.

Using morphological criteria, hepatitis due to either infection with non-A – non-B or hepatitis B cannot be reliably distinguished, and at times, serological tests may not be accurate, since the expression of antibodies against the virus may be altered in an immunocompromised host. Liver function tests (predominantly transaminases), are variably elevated, and can fluctuate.

Sometimes it is difficult to distinguish between viral hepatitis and acute or chronic GVHD. If no other organs are involved, liver biopsy can be helpful in establishing the correct diagnosis and may allow institution of the appropriate therapy. However, the histologic picture in chronic GVHD and chronic hepatitis may be similar, showing bile duct abnormalities along with cholestasis. A high serum alkaline phosphatase is usually more suggestive of chronic GVHD, as this is not a feature of non-A – non-B hepatitis.

Data on prognosis and incidence of hepatitis after marrow transplantation are sparse. In constrast to active hepatitis, HBsAg carrier status does not appear to be a risk factor for posttransplant hepatic complications such as VOD. However, a chronic hepatitis B infection can be exacerbated, during immune reconstitution or by superinfection with the δ-agent.

Cytomegalovirus

Next to non-A – non-B hepatitis, infections with CMV are most frequent. Histopathological alterations include multiple foci of necrosis, portal infiltrates with lymphoid cells, cholestasis and sometimes massive necrosis. Diagnosis can best be obtained through biopsy material. Although giant nuclear and cytoplasmic inclusions are typical, these are sometimes difficult to find. Monoclonal antibodies against CMV antigens together with in situ hybridization techniques may be useful in diagnosing CMV infection. However, in situ hybridization of the CMV genome cannot distinguish between active replication and persistent or latent infection. At present there is no effective treatment for these patients. The inhibitor of viral DNA replication, ganciclovir (DHPG), high dose hyperimmunoglobulin against CMV, and the polymerase inhibitor foscarnet are currently undergoing therapeutic trials.

VZV, HSV

Reactivation of herpes virus occurs in a majority of seropositive patients after transplantation, unless extended prophylaxis with acyclovir is given. The incidence of acute hepatitis related to HSV is not known and can only be estimated. VZV – hepatitis is usually seen late, about 9–12 months post transplant with an incidence of 50–60% in patients with chronic GVHD. If the disease presents without skin involvement, abdominal pain may be the leading symptom, although rare fulminant hepatic failure in the absence of a skin rash can occur. HSV and VZV viruses can be identified by immunofluorescent staining of frozen sections using monoclonal antibodies. If administered promptly, treatment with acyclovir is usually effective.

Adenovirus

Infections with adenovirus generally occur within the first three months of transplantation. Severe acute GVHD has been shown to be a risk factor for invasive infection, including focal hepatic necrosis, and, in an occasional patient, fulminant liver failure. Isolated liver involvement apparently is not common and usually lungs, kidneys and urinary bladder show signs of infection. As with HSV/VZV, diagnosis can best be obtained by immunofluorescent staining of frozen sections with monoclonal antibodies.

Bacterial Infections

Bacterial infections of the liver in the form of abscesses and cholangitis are suprisingly infrequent after marrow grafting presumably due to the early use of broad-spectrum antibiotics. However, with gram negative septicemia concomitant moderate elevations of liver enzymes and bilirubin can occur. This may confound the diagnosis of VOD, acute GVHD, viral infection, or drug induced liver damage which may be present concurrently.

Fungal Infections

Hepatic involvement by fungi occurs in over 50% of patients with disseminated fungal infection. Most commonly, Candida albicans and tropicalis are involved but other species such as Candida parapsilosis, stellatoidea or krusei are found as well. Usually fungal cultures from extrahepatic sites (stool, urine, oropharynx) are positive. Aspergillus species cause a more fulminant clinical picture preferentially involving different organs (lungs, brain, paranasal sinus), and liver involvement is usually documented only at autopsy. As in the general patient population aspergillus does not usually grow from cultures. Other fungi such as Trichosporum cutaneum or Histoplasma capsulatum are found less frequently.

Fungal infections of the liver may present as cysts, granulomas, abscesses and obstruction of biliary ducts by fungus balls. Obstruction of hepatic veins may mimic veno-occlusive disease. Patients often will have persistent fever, liver tenderness and an elevation of alkaline phosphatase. Ultrasound, computed tomography and guided fine needle aspiration should be performed to obtain the diagnosis.

Drug Induced Hepatic Damage

Methotrexate

Although elevations of transaminases are commonly seen after higher doses of intravenous methotrexate, no significant histopathologic changes in the liver have been described with the low dose prophylactic regimen (10–15 mg/m^2 i.v. or i.t.) used in the setting of marrow transplantation. However, in combination with other hepatotoxic drugs, such as cyclosporine, methotrexate may add toxicity and should be withheld if the bilirubin increases significantly.

Cyclosporine

Cyclosporine is extensively metabolized in the liver ($\sim$90%) and subject to biliary elimination. Studies have shown that the serum half-life increases as serum bilirubin increases: in patients with no, mild, and moderate hepatic dysfunction the corresponding half life values were 3.5, 5.8 and 8.7 hours. Serum bilirubin correlates most accurately with cyclosporine elimination. Therefore, it is recommended that cyclosporine intake be reduced if the bilirubin increases, possibly in consultation with the transplant center.

Cyclosporine can induce a *centrilobular hemorrhagic necrosis,* and the simultaneous administration of cyclosporine along with preparative chemoradiotherapy can increase liver toxicity. This particular observation was made in patients with aplastic anemia who developed severe VOD when cyclosporine was given during the pretransplant preparative period.

Observations in renal transplant patients, in whom no GVHD is expected, indicate that cyclosporine frequently causes a moderate rise in bilirubin and, less often, transaminases. Alkaline phosphatase may be only slightly elevated. A similar pattern is observed in marrow transplant recipients. When cyclosporine is started on the day before transplantation, a slight increase in bilirubin (2–3 mg%) is often seen during the first week after marrow infusion. Usually other liver tests (transaminases and alkaline phosphatase) remain normal or are only mildly elevated. Differential diagnosis of cyclosporine hepatotoxicity and VOD should not be a problem since VOD usually is associated with characteristic clinical signs (weight gain, tenderness of the liver, ascites) and elevated liver function tests. However, occasionally, both problems can be superimposed.

The incidence of transient liver function abnormalities is higher when cyclosporine and methotrexate are combined. Cyclosporine toxicity can often be distinguished from hepatic GVHD by its onset early posttransplant, the rate of rise of serum bilirubin, and confirmation of high cyclosporine blood levels. However, if liver toxicity develops later, it may be impossible to identify the underlying cause without additional diagnostic procedures.

Azathioprine

This drug has been used to treat active chronic GVHD, and is still given to patients who are resistant to other therapy. Azathioprine can cause an increase in alkaline phosphatase and transaminases. The chemical abnormalities of chronic GVHD may resemble those of azathioprine-induced liver toxicity. A liver biopsy may be helpful and findings such as bile duct lesions or ductopenia are more consistent with chronic GVHD.

Parenteral Nutrition

Parenteral nutrition can cause cholestatic hepatitis and hepatomegaly due to fatty changes and water accumulation. Jaundice is usually mild and liver function tests may be slightly elevated. Due to a lack of regular gallbladder contractions, dilatation of the bladder and bile stasis can occur in these patients. This can lead to *acalculous cholecystitis,* and occasionally obstruction of the cystic duct, manifested in the form of biliary colic.

Recurrent Malignancy

Although a rare event, this possibility should be considered particularly in patients transplanted for the treatment of malignant lymphoma. Usually ultrasound, computed tomography and liver biopsy are helpful in obtaining the diagnosis quickly.

References

Beschorner WE, Pino J, Boitnott JK, Tutschka RJ, Santos GW (1980) Pathology of the liver with bone marrow transplantation. Effect of busulfan, carmustine, acute graft versus host disease and cytomegalovirus infection. Am J Pathol 99: 396

Deeg HJ, Shulman HM, Schmidt E, Yee GC, Thomas ED, Storb R (1986) Marrow graft rejection and veno-occlusive disease of the liver in patients with aplastic anemia conditioned with cyclophosphamide and cyclosporine. Transplantation 42: 497

Dulley FL, Kanfer EJ, Appelbaum FR, Amos D, Hill RS, Buckner CD, Shulman HH, McDonald GB, Thomas ED (1987) Venocclusive disease of the liver after chemoradiotherapy and autologous bone marrow transplantation. Transplantation 43: 870

Marrie TJ, McDonald ATJ, Coneu PE, Boadreau SFJ (1985) Herpes simplex hepatitis – use of immunoperoxidase to demonstrate the viral antigen in hepatocytes. Gastroenterology 82: 71

McDonald GB, Sharma P, Matthews DE, Shulman HM, Thomas ED (1985) The clinical course of 53 patients with veno-occlusive disease of the liver after marrow transplantation. Transplantation 39: 603

McDonald GB, Sharma P, Matthews DE, Shulman HM, Thomas ED (1984) Venoocclusive disease of the liver after bone marrow transplantation: diagnosis, incidence and predisposing factors. Hepatology 4: 116

McDonald GB, Shulman HM, Sullivan KM, Spencer GD (1986) Intestinal and hepatic complications of human bone marrow transplantation. Part I and II. Gastroenterology 90: 460

Menard DB, Gisselbrecht C, Marty M, Reyes F, Dhumeaux D (1980) Antineoplastic agents and the liver. Gastroenterology 78: 142

Roslyn JJ, Pitt HA, Mann LL et al (1983) Gall bladder disease in patients on long-term parenteral nutrition. Gastroenterology 84: 148

Shulman HM, McDonald GB, Matthews D et al (1980) An analysis of hepatic veno-occlusive disease and centrilobular hepatic degeneration following bone marrow transplantation. Gastroenterology 79: 1178

Snoves DC, Weisdorf, SA, Ramsay NV, McGlave P, Kersey JH (1984) Hepatic graft versus host disease: a study of the predictive value of liver biopsy in diagnosis. Hepatology 4: 123

Wade JC, Gaffey M, Wiernik PH et al (1983) Hepatitis in patients with acute nonlymphoblastic leukemia. Am J Med 75: 413

Yee GC, Kennedy MS, Storb R, Thomas ED (1984) Effect of hepatic dysfunction on oral cyclosporine pharmacokinetics in marrow transplant patients. Blood 64: 1277

7. Urinary Tract

In contrast to the liver, the kidneys are rarely the *primary* target of a pathological event after bone marrow transplantation. GVHD (acute or chronic) does not visibly affect the kidney and a specific disease entity related to radio-chemotherapy damage such as radiation nephritis has not been observed. However, it is likely that a subclinical degree of tubular damage occurs during the conditioning regimen. Renal impairment is predominantly secondary to circulatory disturbances associated with veno-occlusive disease, septicemia or hypovolemic shock. Further some of the drugs frequently used posttransplant can injure the tubular system. The severity of renal impairment can range from mild prerenal insufficiency to acute oliguric (or anuric) renal failure.

Common causes of urinary tract diseases posttransplant include:

- Renal insufficiency secondary to circulatory problems
- Drug induced toxicity
- Infections

Renal Insufficiency Secondary to Circulatory Problems

This disorder is often a consequence of intravascular volume depletion, and associated hypotension. Common causes are capillary leak syndrome, severe gastrointestinal losses and septic shock. In severe cases prerenal insufficiency may lead to acute oliguric renal failure. Treatment should be directed at maintaining sufficient intravascular volume by infusion of albumin and red cells, correction of electrolyte imbalances and dose reduction doses of potentially nephrotoxic drugs such as cyclosporine, amphotericin B and aminoglycoside antibiotics (see below).

Prerenal insufficiency due to circulatory imbalance has to be distinguished from a catabolic state which usually shows a disproportional rise of serum urea compared to relatively normal serum creatinine. If renal function abnormalities are due to a severe catabolic state, proteins and dietary calories should be given freely which, however, should be restricted in prerenal insufficiency.

In severe cases of prerenal insufficiency or toxic damage *acute renal failure* secondary to acute tubular necrosis can develop, in particular when nephrotoxic drugs are given at the same time. Most of these patients will have a high output failure with subsequent oliguria. Common causes include nephrotoxins (such as cyclosporine, aminoglycosides, amphotericin B), prolonged hypotension or the hepatorenal syndrome in the course of severe veno-occlusive disease. Some patients may require temporary dialysis. Because of the high protein requirement of patients after transplantation, amino acids should be administered routinely. Nonprotein calories can be supplied by concentrated dextrose (ie. 35% or greater) and lipids. Furthermore, it is advisable to keep the hemoglobin of a high level (> 100 g/l) to provide sufficient oxygen to the kidney and to increase the intravascular osmotic pressure. Although somewhat controversial, most centers also give low doses of continuous dopamine infusion (2 µg/kg/min). The prognosis of renal impairment secondary to prerenal insufficiency is usually rather good. After the underlying disease has been corrected with appropriate drug dose adjustment and supportive measures, kidney function can recover completely.

Drug Induced Renal Toxicity

Although several antineoplastic drugs, such as CCNU, mitomycin and adriamycin, are nephrotoxic, no significant nephrotoxicity has been associated with drugs commonly used for the preparative regimen before marrow grafting. However, they might cause sub-threshold damage to the kidney which can lead to exaggerated responses with other agents. Most of the potentially nephrotoxic drugs such as cyclosporine, various antibiotic, antifungal and antiviral agents are employed in the posttransplant period.

Aminoglycosides. Aminoglycosides are frequently given after bone marrow transplantation as treatment or prophylaxis of infections with gram negative bacteria. However, they are nephrotoxic in a dose related fashion as they accumulate in the liposomes of proximal tubular cells, where they are bound to phospholipids. This may lead to mostly reversible focal necrosis and interstitial proliferation. The degree of nephrotoxicity seems to vary between different aminoglycosides and it appears that amikacin is the least nephrotoxic compound.

Cyclosporine. Nephrotoxicity of cyclosporine is associated with renal vascular injury, most likely due to inhibition of prostacyclin synthesis in the epithelial vascular cells. Histologically vascular injury with arteriolar and glomerular capillary thrombosis as well as interstitial sclerosis have been seen. Early signs of kidney damage by cyclosporine can consist of proteinuria, bicarbonate loss, impaired urinary concentrating ability and urinary casts.

Some renal function impairment during cyclosporine treatment can be expected in nearly every patient. About 50% of all patients will develop an elevated serum creatinine level ≥ 50% above baseline within days or weeks of starting cyclosporine. Volume depletion, additional nephrotoxic drugs, hepatic dysfunction (especially veno-occlusive disease), septicemia and prolonged hypotension are associated with a more rapid rise in creatinine. Particularly aminoglycosides and amphotericin B given concurrently with cyclosporine can increase nephrotoxicity significantly. The same is true for trimethoprim-sulfamethoxazole, as it interferes with tubular secretion of creatinine. Renal dysfunction is usually reversible after withdrawal of cyclosporine, even in patients who have had elevated serum creatinine levels for several months. However, if severe renal damage has occured, recovery might not be complete and chronic renal damage may persist.

In some patients treated with cyclosporine, a syndrome reminiscent of the hemolytic-uremic syndrome with renal insufficiency has been reported. The pathogenesis is largely unknown. Drug induced endothelial injury is suspected with subsequent fragmentation of red cells and release of procoagulant material with concomitant coagulation disorder.

If renal dysfunction develops in patients on cyclosporine therapy, some drug adjustments are recommended:

1. When creatinine rises markedly (50% over previous day's value) 1–2 doses of cyclosporine should be withheld, hydration should be increased and other nephrotoxins should be discontinued, if possible.
2. When creatinine rises gradually, the dosage should be reduced by at least 25%. In general, it is advisable to give the drug at reduced level rather than to withhold it.
3. If the creatinine is between 1.5 mg/dl and 2.0 mg/dl (132–177 μmol/l), the daily dose should be reduced by 50%.
4. If the creatinine exceeds 2.0 mg/dl (177 μmol/l), cyclosporine should be held.

The role of cyclosporine levels in monitoring drug related renal toxicity is not yet entirely clear. Even high blood levels over a long period of time are not necessarily associated with significant renal impairment. This is particularly true for patients who also have hypertriglyceridemia. In these patients fairly high cyclosporine levels have been observed without any renal impairment. It is presumed that the drug is bound primarily to lipoproteins and that, therefore, the free unbound fraction of the drug may actually be low. Many investigators agree that careful monitoring of serum creatinine and blood urea nitrogen levels as indicators of renal damage requiring adjustment of cyclosporine dose is the most practical approach.

Acyclovir. Renal damage can occur when acyclovir is given intravenously at higher doses. Crystal formation in the renal tubules, the collecting ducts or both have been described. When the drug is administered by slow infusion over one hour along with adequate hydration, the incidence of raised blood urea nitrogen and creatinine levels should be lower. However, if renal failure develops in a transplant patient and creatinine clearance is below 50 ml/min, an acyclovir dose reduction is required. The same is true for ganciclovir (DHGP) used experimentally for prophylaxis and treatment of cytomegalovirus infections.

Cyclophosphamide – Cystitis. Hemorrhagic cystitis is the most frequent serious side effect of high dose cyclophosphamide therapy in marrow transplant patients. It is caused by the urotoxic metabolite of cyclophosphamide, acrolein. The incidence of this complication can be reduced by forced diuresis (200–250 ml/hr in adults) with or without bladder irradigation. Nonetheless, about 30% will develop cystitis despite these preventive measures. Another approach is to give mesna (2-mercaptoethane sulfonate sodium) concomitant with the cyclophosphamide infusion. Mesna is administered intravenously (160% of the cyclophosphamide dose), and rapidly excreted via the urinary tract. Within the urinary tract, mesna combines with acrolein to form a non-toxic compound. Mesna reduces the incidence of hemorrhagic cystitis by about 50%. However, the timing of mesna administration is important (before cyclophosphamide, then 3 h, 6 h and 9 h after cyclophosphamide or alternatively as a continuous infusion), and timing errors may result in a loss of its protective effect.

It appears that treatment with busulphan prior to transplantation, mostly given to patients with chronic myelogenous leukemia, also increases the risk of developing hemorrhagic cystitis.

Apart from cyclophosphamide, etoposide at higher doses can cause hemorrhagic cystitis which, however, can be prevented by forced diuresis for at least three days after etoposide has been stopped.

Treatment options for hemorrhagic cystitis are limited. Recently the use of intravesical prostaglandin E_2 has been reported to be successful in some patients. Vigorous continuous hydration should be given. Some patients may require cauterization of bleeding mucosa via cystoscopy.

It should be pointed out that the course of hemorrhagic cystitis can vary greatly. Some patients experience a short period of hematuria following chemotherapy administration. In others, it occurs with some time lag and may manifest itself, for example, when the patient develops severe thrombocytopenia. Delayed problems after resolution of the acute cystitis are rare. However, an occasional patient may develop bladder spasms and may be plagued by reduced bladder capacity.

Infections

In general, infectious complications of the kidney are not very frequent after marrow transplantation. Particularly, bacterial renal infections such as pyelonephritis are rarely encountered. Kidney involvement often occurs as part of a systemic infection, and renal impairment can develop as a consequence of bacteremia and septic shock. About 7% of autopsied marrow recipients show involvement of the kidney with fungus. The most common organisms found are Candida species. Abscess formation has been described.

Viral infections: Systemic CMV infection can also affect the kidney. However, changes are nonspecific and it is not clear whether or not they have functional consequences. As described above, cyclophosphamide-induced cystitis usually becomes manifest within the first days of infusion of the drug, and may persist for up to 2 months. If hemorrhagic cystitis develops later after marrow transplantation, other causes specifically infections of viral etiology must be considered. In a series of about 1,000 transplanted patients, adenovirus could be isolated from the urine of 10% of patients. One quarter of infected patients had decreased renal function (serum creatinine > 2 mg/dl (177 μmol/l)), and all but one required hemodialysis. About the same number of patients presented with cystitis. Of these, however, only half showed positive urine cultures for adenovirus. Most

patients with adenovirus infection also have signs of disseminated disease involving organs such as lung, gut and liver.
Histologic changes diagnostic of adenovirus infection in the kidneys include viral inclusions associated with tubular epithelial necrosis, interstitial inflammation and hemorrhage. The majority of patients with adenovirus infection may have graft-versus-host disease at the same time. Interestingly, isolation of patients in laminar airflow rooms does not prevent infection with adenovirus suggesting an endogenous source.
Besides adenovirus, polyomaviruses have been associated with late onset hemorrhagic cystitis. Nearly one third of all transplanted patients excrete the virus in the urine. It is not yet clear whether the virus can also cause infections of other organs such as lung or liver. In some patients, hepatic dysfunction has been suspected to be caused by polyomavirus. Cytomegalovirus can cause severe and often fatal infections of the lung and liver. For unknown reasons, cytomegalovirus does not primarily affect the kidney although urinary excretion is not infrequent.
Treatment options for adeno- and polyomavirus infections are limited. If the patient is receiving postgrafting immunosuppression, and acute GVHD is not active, a dose reduction of immunosuppressive drugs might be considered. In addition, polyvalent immunoglobulins intravenously can be given since these preparations generally contain antiviral titers. It should be noted, however, that no data is available as to the efficacy of these measures.

References

Gerrera GA, Alexander RW, Cooley CF et al (1986) Cytomegalovirus glomerulopathy: A controversial lesion. Kidney 29: 725

Kennedy MS, Deeg HJ, Siegel M, Crowley JJ, Storb R, Thomas ED (1983) Acute renal toxicity with combined use of amphotericin B and cyclosporine after marrow transplantation. Transplantation 35: 211

Nemunaitis J, Deeg HJ, Yee GC (1986) High cyclosporine levels after bone marrow transplantation associated with hypertriglyceridemia. Lancet II: 744

Palestine AG, Austin HA III, Balow JE, et al (1986) Renal histopathologic alterations in patients treated with cyclosporine for uveitis. N Eng J Med 314: 1293

Shields AF, Hackman RC, Fife KH, Corey L, Meyers JD (1985) Adenovirus infections in patients undergoing bone marrow transplantation. N Eng J Med 312: 529

Shulman H, Striker G, Deeg HJ, Kennedy M, Storb R, Thomas ED (1981) Nephrotoxicity of cyclosporine A after allogeneic bone marrow transplantation: glomerular thrombosis and tubular injury. N Eng J Med 305: 1392

Thomas AE, Patterson J, Prentice HG, et al (1987) Haemorrhagic cystitis in bone marrow transplantation patients: possible increased risk associated with busulphan therapy. Bone Marrow Transplant 1: 347

8. Central Nervous System (CNS)

The spectrum of CNS complications after marrow grafting is notable for lack of direct involvement of the brain, in contrast to many other organs by GVHD. The following major CNS complications have been observed after transplantation:
- Leucoencephalopathy
- Drug toxicity
- Infection
- Hemorrhage
- Recurrent malignancy

Since the symptomatology of these different entities is often very similar, a lumbar puncture almost always has to be performed to help establish the correct diagnosis. Specimens of the cerebrospinal fluid should be examined for:
1. number and type of cells, and presence of micro-organisms (gram stains for bacteria, silver and india ink stains for fungus, and Ziehl Neelson for Mycobacterium tuberculosis),
2. protein and sugar,
3. bacteriologic cultures, virus isolation and cryptococcal antigen.

Before a lumbar puncture can be safely performed, a low platelet count has to be corrected, and usually at least $30 \times 10^9/l$ platelets are recommended. Furthermore, a lumbar puncture carries some risk if the pressure of the cerebrospinal fluid is high, for it increases the possibility of a fatal cerebellar or tentorial pressure cone. Therefore, a CT-scan of the brain as a first diagnostic measure should be obtained.

Leukoencephalopathy

Pathogenesis

The combined application of CNS irradiation at doses of 20 Gy or above, and intrathecal chemotherapy, specifically methotrexate, can result in irreversible brain damage. Both modalities act synergistically in the sense that radiation apparently changes the blood-brain barrier and allows the intrathecal drug improved access to the central nervous system. Intrathecal methotrexate has most often been described as being associated with the development of the disease.

The role of intrathecal cytarabine in the development of leukoencephalopathy is not yet clear, probably because it has been given less often along with radiation than methotrexate. However, considering the potential neurotoxic effects of this drug, a similar frequency of leukoencephalopathic changes as with methotrexate can be anticipated.

Histopathology

Demyelinization is accompanied by multifocal to confluent non-inflammatory necrosis; furthermore, dystrophic calcification and ventricular dilatation can be seen.
Risk factors for the development of leukoencephalopathy include:
- Pretransplant CNS therapy or prophylaxis with irradiation, intrathecal chemotherapy or both,
- Preparative regimen containing total body irradiation,
- More than 5 courses of intrathecal methotrexate post transplant.

After marrow transplantation, leukoencephalopathy is seen almost exclusively in patients with acute lymphoblastic leukemia who have received cranial or craniospinal irradiation or intrathecal chemotherapy, or both before preparation for marrow transplantation. In such patients, the risk of developing leukoencephalopathy is about 7%. The conditioning regimen by itself, and posttransplant methotrexate do not appear to increase the risk of this complication in children who have not previously been given CNS prophylaxis or therapy.

The manifestations of leukoencephalopathy are not age related. The fact that it is more often seen in young patients might be related to the age distribution of acute lymphoblastic leukemia. Data from a large patient population have shown that 3 of 7 transplanted patients were over the age of 20. There is evidence that a lower dose of posttransplant methotrexate administered via an Ommaya reservoir may avoid neurotoxicity.

Despite the occurence of leukoencephalopathy the overall risk of developing this complication is lower than the risk of CNS relapse when posttransplant intrathecal methotrexate is omitted. In one study among patients with a history of CNS disease, the probability of CNS relapse was 52% if they did not receive intrathecal methotrexate compared to 17% if the posttransplant prophylaxis was given. For patients who had *no* CNS disease before marrow grafting, the corresponding figures were 19% and 4% respectively.

Diagnosis

Symptoms can be nonspecific such as: lethargy, slurred speech, ataxia, seizures, confusion, dysphagia, spasticity, dementia and decerebrate posturing. Computed tomograms of the brain may show, as an early sign, a decreased density, which may be reversible, and later, destruction of the white matter, ventricular dilatation and calcification. Myelin basic protein and enolase levels are elevated in the CNS fluid during the acute phase and recent data suggest that they may be used to monitor patients at high risk of developing leukoencephalopathy. Nuclear magnetic resonance imaging may establish diagnosis of cerebral lesions earlier and more reliably than is possible with conventional CT-scanning.

Clinical Course

Symptoms of leukoencephalopathy usually become manifest during the first month after transplantation and may include a spectrum of nonspecific neurological changes such as confusion, seizures and paraplegia, which can progress to a severe irreversible clinical picture. From experience with conventional treatment of leukemia, it is known that early leukoencephalopathy-associated changes may be reversible when chemoradiotherapy of the brain is stopped in time. However, no such information is available for transplanted patients.

A delayed form of neurotoxicity may become obvious later (months to years) after marrow grafting. Histopathology shows white matter necrosis and dystrophic calcification of the small vessels. Symptoms are forgetfulness, confusion and poor performance at school, specifically, difficulties with reading and arithmetic. This is most often seen in patients who received combined radiation/intrathecal methrotrexate before they were three years old.

Differential diagnosis

Meningeal involvement of leukemia can create a block of cerebrospinal fluid drainage and may cause symptoms and signs of increased intracranial pressure. CT-scanning and lumbar puncture usually establish the diagnosis, and help to differentiate leukoencephalopathy from infectious and bleeding complications of the brain.

Treatment

Leukoencephalopathy is a degenerative process, and no effective therapy is available. Therefore prevention of this complication should be attempted. One can, for instance, consider alternative conditioning regimens not including total body irradiation for patients at risk. Possibly determination of myelin basic protein in cerebrospinal fluid can identify patients at risk. In any case, no more than five doses of intrathecal methotrexate should be given after transplantation, since recent data suggest that there is no added benefit from more than five doses irrespective of CNS leukemia status at transplantation.

Recurrence of Malignancy

CNS recurrence of malignancy is relatively infrequent in patients given a marrow transplant for acute myelogenous leukemia or chronic myelogenous leukemia in chronic phase. However, it does occur in a fraction of patients transplanted for acute lymphoblastic leukemia or some high risk lymphomas. In these patients CNS relapse often heralds bone marrow relapse.

The probability of developing CNS relapse after marrow transplantation in patients with *acute myelogenous leukemia* in remission is less than 2%. In contrast, patients with *acute lymphoblastic leukemia* have a 38% probability of recurrent disease if no intrathecal prophylaxis is given posttransplant. Therefore, for these patients posttransplant methotrexate is recommended regardless of previous chemoradiotherapy of the brain and spine. Apparently there is no added benefit from more than five doses of posttransplant methotrexate or cytosine arabinoside irrespective of CNS leukemia status at transplant. Table 21 summarizes the current recommendation of CNS prophylaxis after marrow grafting for various malignancies.

Prevention of the often irreversible disease can be achieved by lowering the dose of prophylactic radiation to 18 Gy. Similarly, if possible, checking the pharmacokinetics of methotrexate in the patient's cerebrospinal fluid may help to detect abnormally elevated methotrexate levels. Furthermore, reduced doses of intrathecal methotrexate should be given to children under the age of two.

Neurological symptoms of CNS malignancy are usually nonspecific and analysis of cerebrospinal fluid and CT-scanning can help to distinguish CNS relapse from infectious or bleeding complications.

Table 21. Intrathecal Methotrexate After Marrow Transplantation

Diagnosis:
- Acute Myelogenous Leukemia – remission or relapse
- Chronic Myelogenous Leukemia in chronic phase or blast crisis of myeloid type
- Hodgkin's Disease
- Non-Hodgkin's lymphoma, low grade histology

  Recommendations:
  - Diagnostic lumbar puncture pre-transplant, and injection of one dose of methotrexate
  - If cerebrospinal fluid negative for leukemia cells no further methotrexate will be given
  - If evidence of leukemia, one additional dose of methotrexate pretransplant and four doses posttransplant

Diagnosis:
- Acute Lymphoblastic Leukemia – remission or relapse
- Chronic Myelogenous Leukemia – blast crisis of lymphoid type
- Non-Hodgkin's Lymphoma, aggressive histology

  Recommendations:
  - Diagnostic lumbar puncture pre-transplant, and injection of one dose of methotrexate
  - If cerebrospinal fluid negative for leukemic cells no further intrathecal methotrexate pre-grafting; if positive one additional dose of methotrexate will be given
  - All patients to be given four doses of intrathecal methotrexate post transplant

Infections of the CNS

Fungus

Aspergillus

The most frequent infections of the CNS, are due to fungi. CNS involvement in the form of brain abscess is relatively common in patients who have disseminated aspergillosis. Aspergillus species are primarily respiratory pathogens, and consequently, the majority of infections involve either the sinus or the lungs. In about 30 percent, however, the infection disseminates throughout the body since aspergillus has a propensity for invading blood vessels. The rhino-cerebrae form of aspergillus originates in the sinuses and progresses through soft tissues, cartilage, and bone, causing lesions in the palate and the nose. Occasionally, the infection progresses through the base of the skull to involve the brain. Amphotericin B is the only antifungal agent with established activity against Aspergillus species. It has been combined with 5-fluorocytosine and rifampin, but there is no conclusive evidence that these combinations have any advantages over amphotericin B alone.

Unfortunately, in most cases, even this drug is not capable of controlling the disease, and surgical resection of the abscess is required, a procedure which cannot be performed in most cases of brain abscess.

Candida

Hematogenous dissemination of Candida (Candida albicans, tropicalis, krusei), may manifest with retinal abscesses (symptoms: orbital pain, blurred vision, scotoma, opacities). Meningitis and brain abscesses occur in about 20 percent of patients with disseminated infection. The diagnosis may be difficult to establish because only nonspecific abnormalities may be found in the cerebrospinal fluid, and the fungus may not be seen or successfully cultured.

Cryptococcosis

Unlike candidiasis and aspergillosis, cryptococcosis is aquired prior to hospitalization. The organism is ubiquitous in animals and soil specimens. Infections begin in the lungs where, in normal persons, it may remain asymptomatic and resolve without therapy. Dissemination can occur in patients after marrow transplantation and central nervous system infection is a regular feature which may manifest as meningoencephalitis. Early manifestations include headache, nausea, staggering gait, irritability, confusion, and blurred vision. Both fever and nuchal rigidity are usually mild or absent. A chest X-ray may disclose a dense infiltrate if pulmonary cryptococcosis is present at the same time. Primary lesions are present in about 10% of patients. A lumbar puncture is the most useful test, and an India ink smear may reveal encapsulated yeast. A test for cryptococcal antigen may be positive. The most definitive test, however, is the culture.

Bacteria

Meningitis due to bacteria is, overall, rare and may occur later on after marrow grafting, predominantly in recipients who have developed chronic GVHD. Pneumococcus, meningococcus, hemophilus influenzae and klebsiella pneumoniae are the most common pathogens. The manifestation are those of any acute pyogenic meningitis and include chills, fever, headache, nuchal rigidity, delirium and cranial nerve palsies. Occasionally brain abscesses from staphylococcus aureus are seen. If bacterial infection of the CNS is suspected, spinal fluid should be investigated. With appropriate chemotherapy, recovery can be expected in ⅔ of all cases.

Viruses

Viral infections of the CNS are infrequent after marrow grafting. Many patients are placed on prophylactic acyclovir after transplantation and, therefore, CNS infections with herpes virus are uncommon. However, specifically in patients who are not receiving prophylaxis with acyclovir, or in those with chronic GVHD, herpes simplex (HSV) or disseminated varicella zoster infection can be the cause of encephalitis which may present with a range of neurological complications. HSV type I can ascend from the respiratory epithelium of the nose up the olfactory tract to reach the frontal and temporal areas of the brain. In the cerebrospinal fluid, a lymphocytosis and elevated protein content may be found as fairly nonspecific alterations. Early diagnosis can best be obtained by nuclear magnetic resonance in combination with electroencephalogram. Usually, a computed tomogram of the brain will not show signs of focal necrosis before the third day of infection. The only definitive means of diagnosing HSV encephalitis is the isolation of HSV by brain biopsy. Treatment with acyclovir 10 mg/kg three times daily can be effective when started in time before the onset of coma, and full recovery may occur.

Toxoplasmosis

Reactivation of quiescent infection (cysts) with liberation of toxoplasmosis trophozoites may occur virtually anywhere throughout the body. However, about 50% of transplanted patients with fatal toxoplasmosis have signs and symptoms of encephalitis and more than 90% also have pathological evidence of brain involvement. Neurological signs can be highly variable and may include: disturbances of consciousness, motor impairment, diffuse meningoencephalitis, cerebellar ataxia and seizures.

Serologic tests may be insensitive in patients lacking immune response. However, toxoplasma gondii can be isolated from the peripheral buffy coat cells and inoculated on human fibroblast cultures. A cytopathic effect is seen in an infected individual after 2–3 weeks. In addition, CNS fluid can have some characteristic features such as mononuclear pleocytosis and pronounced elevation in protein along with normal glucose. For treatment, pyrimethamin should be given with a loading dose of 2 mg/kg for the first two days. In severe infections, doses can be doubled and given every day. In addition, sulfadiazine is recommended in a dose of 100 mg/kg/day.

Hemorrhage

Hemorrhagic complications of the CNS are not very frequent since patients are usually given prophylactic platelet support to maintain a level of about 20,000/mm^3. Even in allosensitized recipients, a low platelet count is frequently tolerated without hemorrhage as these younger individuals are not expected to have an underlying degenerative process of the vascular system. However, the situation is different if the patient is septic and has concomitant coagulation abnormalities. In an occasional patient, hemorrhage may also be seen as a complication of CNS fungal infection, most often aspergillus. In any event, CT-scan of the brain along with a lumbar puncture will allow the diagnosis to be obtained quickly.

Drug Induced Neurotoxicity

The spectrum of drugs used before and after marrow grafting that can cause neurotoxicity is limited.

Cytosine arabinoside (Ara C). High dose Ara C (1.5–3 g/m^2 for several days) is part of various preparative protocols. Beside hepatotoxicity, neuropathy is a serious complication which has to be separated from leukoencephalopathy, infection, bleeding and leukemia of the CNS. Histologically one can see damage or loss of Purkinje cells from the lateral hemisphere along with proliferation of astrocytes. Since about 40–60% of the Ara C plasma concentration can be found in the cerebrospinal fluid, and CNS toxicity is related to the dose administered, and not to the duration of exposure, the incidence of CNS symptoms increases significantly at a cumulative dose of over 36 g/m^2. However, occasional symptoms may develop at lower doses if the patient has been treated with high dose Ara C before transplantation, eg. during remission induction therapy. Symptoms usually develop within 6–8 days after the first dose and may include personality changes, disturbances in the level of consciousness, headache, somnolence, confusion, scomatoma, paraplegia, cerebellar toxicity, and occasionally seizures. Symptoms are reversible within a few days after stopping the drug. However, cerebellar ataxia and dysarthria might be irreversible in about 10% of all patients.

Cyclosporine. Patients on this drug can present with a variety of neurological symptoms listed in Table 22. In a recent series, about 8 percent of patients treated with cyclosporine experienced neurological illnesses. These included quadriparesis, urinary retention, ataxia, drowsiness and mental confusion. Some of the neurological symptoms (in particular grand mal and focal seizures, tremor, depression and cerebellar ataxia) have been linked to a low level of serum magnesium which is caused by renal wasting secondary to cyclosporine induced tubular damage. Regular magnesium replacement may prevent these neurological

Table 22. Neurotoxicity of Cyclosporine

Tremor
Mental Confusion
Muscle Weakness
Paraesthesia
Seizures (grand mal)
Transverse Myelitis
Quadriparesis
Cerebellar Ataxia
Drowsiness

complications. However, not all neurological side effects are clearly linked to a low magnesium level. This is particularly true for patients who develop grand mal seizures. There is also no clear link to an elevated plasma or serum cyclosporine level. In some cases, the concurrent administration of high dose methylprednisolone has been suspected to be causative. Children seem to be more susceptible to the toxic neurological effects (in particular fits) of cyclosporine. It has also been suggested that cyclosporine neurotoxicity is more often seen in patients transplanted for a hematologic malignancy, but, rarely in patients who have received a transplant for aplastic anemia. It may be possible that the neurotoxicity is cumulative with cyclosporine, intrathecal methotrexate and total body irradiation all contributing. However, if high dose methylprednisolone is given concurrently, convulsions have also been described in patients transplanted for aplastic anemia. Therefore, if a patient is on cyclosporine prophylaxis and requires additional anti-graft versus host disease medication in the form of high dose methylprednisolone, some centers recommend that Dilantin (phenytoin) at a dose of 100 mg three times daily for that time period be administered after an appropriate loading dose. It should be noted, however, that clearance of cyclosporine by the liver and kidney is increased by dilantin or phenobarbital in contrast to ketoconazole and cimetidine, which decrease cyclosporine clearance.

Tremor is rather common in patients on cyclosporine and not predictive of any further neurological side effect. In some patients, grand mal tremor of the upper extremities can occur. In an occasional patient, mental depression might be the only sign of cyclosporine neurotoxicity and disappears when the drug is stopped.

Descriptions of the pathological changes associated with cyclosporine neurotoxicity are sparse. Cyclosporine, however, plays a role in the pathogenesis of vascular lesions by inhibiting vascular prostacyclin synthesis. This may lead to microthrombi and focal necrosis. There are some case reports implicating a disturbance of the blood-brain barrier due to cyclosporine leading to bile staining edema and focal necrosis of the brain.

Acyclovir. Approximately 1% of patients receiving intravenous acyclovir can develop encephalopathic changes characterized by either lethargy, obtundation, tremors, confusion, hallucinations, agitation, seizures or coma. Therefore, acyclovir should be used with caution in patients who have shown neurologic side effects to other neurotoxic drugs (eg. cytosine-arabinoside, cyclosporine) or those receiving intrathecal methotrexate at the same time. The potential neurotoxic effects of acyclovir seem to be correlated to be dose administered and therefore, treatment using doses higher that 200 mg/m^2 three times daily should be carefully monitored for neurotoxic side effects.

Steroids. Steroids are part of most prophylactic and therapeutic protocols for acute and chronic GVHD. Side effects are dependent on the size of the dose and the duration of the treatment. Neurological complications can manifest as headache, psychosis, vertigo, convulsions and increased intracranial pressure (pseudotumor cerebri).

References

Atkinson K, Biggs J, Darveniza P, Boland Concannon A, Dobbs A (1984) Cyclosporine-associated central nervous system toxicity after allogeneic bone marrow transplantation. Transplantation 38: 34

Barrett AJ, Kendra JR, Lucas CF, et al (1985) Disturbance of blood-brain barrier after bone marrow transplantation. Lancet II: 280

Lazarus HM, Herzig RH, Herzig GP, Phillips GL, Roessman U, Fishman DJ (1981) Central nervous system toxicity of high-dose systemic cytosine arabinoside. Cancer 48: 2577

Shepp DH, Hackman RC, Conley FK, Anderson JB, Meyers JD (1985) Toxoplasma gondii reactivation identified by detection of parasitemia in tissue culture. Ann Int Med 103: 218

Thompson CB, Sanders JE, Flournoy N, Buckner ED, Thomas ED (1986) The risk of central nervous system relapse and leukoencephalopathy in patients receiving marrow transplants for acute leukemia. Blood 67: 195

Wade JC, Meyers JC (1983) Neurologic symptoms associated with parenteral acyclovir treatment after marrow transplantation. Ann Int Med 98: 921

V. Delayed Transplant Related Problems

1. Follow-up after Discharge from the Transplant Center

Patients who are being discharged from a transplant center to return to the care of their primary physician usually look back on a period of at least 3–4 months of intensive medical and psychological care. Being "discharged" for many patients is frightening and they cope by regressing. Many indeed will state that this moment feels like being reborn; they don't know what is waiting for them in the new world outside.

Every transplant team has developed its' own approach to these problems. However, certain principles apply everywhere. It will have to be clear from the start of the procedure that bone marrow transplantation is not equivalent to being placed in an isolation chamber for life. The patient must have a clear understanding that transplantation is only aimed at cure and never at palliation. Consequently, once the procedure has been completed there will have to be a return to a normal life style. The fact that this treatment is not successful in all patients should not detract from the intent. The aim of any bone marrow transplant be it allogeneic, syngeneic or autologous, is to return the patient to a normal productive life. To allow for a smooth transition from the protected environment of a transplant unit to daily routine on the outside will require a sensitive approach by physicians, nurses, social workers and other support staff. This transition will begin at the transplant center and will continue under the care of the patient's referring physician.

While being cared for at a transplant unit, the patient will have been seen by physicians or nurses at least once or twice weekly after discharge and occasionally every day. Generally a thorough evaluation is carried out before the patient is discharged from the transplant center about three months after transplantation (Table 23). It is recommended that after discharge home the patient be seen at

Table 23. Studies For Longterm Evaluation

– Physical Examination	– Gynecological Evaluation
– Complete Blood Count	– Endocrinologic Evaluation
– Chemistry Survey	Growth Hormone
– Creatinine Clearance	Thyroid Function
– Chest Radiograph	Sex Hormones
– Ophthalmologic Evaluation	– Pulmonary Function Tests
– Oral Medicine Evaluation	

Table 24. Delayed Complications of BMT

– Chronic Graft-vs-Host Disease	– Impaired Growth and Development
– Infections	– Cataracts
– Chronic Pulmonary Disease	– Autoimmune Disorders
– Infertility	– Secondary Malignancies

least once weekly for the first month. If no new medical problems develop and the patient is stable these intervals can be lengthened to two weeks for the next two months, and eventually to three weeks or monthly intervals depending on the patient's clinical status. It appears useful to obtain a chest x-ray at the time the patient is first seen at home, and to monitor liver function tests, complete blood counts as well as food intake and weight regularly. Numerous complications (Table 24) have been observed within months or years of transplantation, and consequently patients require close longterm observation.

Immune function and daily activities. High doses of chemotherapy and total body irradiation given at the time of bone marrow transplantation are intended not only to eradicate the patient's underlying disease but also to suppress the patient's immune system such that the donor marrow can successfully engraft. Consequently, all transplant recipients are subject to a prolonged period of immunodeficiency which is most severe during the first three to four months after transplantation. At the time the patient is discharged home from the transplant center, the period of highest risk of bacterial, fungal and viral infections has been overcome. However, it will take at least 5–6 months, even in patients who do not have any serious complications such as the development of chronic GVHD for immune functions to gradually improve and return to normal.

Thus, the major concern after the patient's discharge is that of infection. Many transplant teams, therefore, recommend that the patient continue to wear a surgical mask for at least six months after transplant. This is aimed at reducing the risk of infections due to certain microorganisms, fungal spores, and pollen. It is likely, however, that the screening effect of these masks is minimal. Nevertheless, these masks appear to be useful to patients as a reminder of the fact that their own immune function has not yet returned to normal, and that they are constantly at risk of infection. It is important for patients to avoid contact with people suffering from viral infections such as measles, German measles, chicken pox, and varicella zoster. Hand washing may be more important than wearing the face mask.

Although most viral infections occur during the first 2–3 months after transplant, some can occur later. Varicella zoster infection is observed in approximately half of all bone marrow transplant recipients within the first year of grafting. This can represent a reactivation of endogenous virus or de novo exogenous infection. If the infection is localized to one or two dermatomes close observation with supportive care and symptomatic treatment appears to be sufficient. If dissemination occurs anti-viral therapy, for example, with vidarabine

(10 mg/kg four times a day) or acyclovir (30 mg/kg in 3 divided doses daily for 7 days) should be given. Although acyclovir may be advantageous in patients with suppressed marrow function, especially platelet counts, there is an approximately 10–20% risk of recurrence of the disease, which is observed only rarely in patients treated with vidarabine. For patients who have inadvertently been exposed to shingles or chicken pox within the first year of transplantation and have not had a recent infection, varicella/zoster immune globulin (ZIG) should be given, starting within six days of exposure. Usually ZIG can be obtained via the Red Cross or other regional blood centers.

Interstitial pneumonia, like other viral infections, usually occurs within the first 2–3 months after transplantation. Most frequently this is caused by cytomegalovirus (CMV). There is no standard proven therapy for this disease. However, there is some recent evidence that the combined use of high dose gancyclovir and intravenous gammaglobulin may be beneficial. Interstitial pneumonitis can also be due to Pneumocystis carinii, although this form is rarely observed in patients on trimethoprim/sulfamethoxazole prophylaxis. Often no causative organism can be identified and such cases are termed idiopathic. Many investigators treat idiopathic interstitial pneumonitis with high dose glucocorticoids (16 mg/kg/day of methylprednisolone), although there are no controlled data proving the efficacy of this treatment. If a patient develops a clinical picture of respiratory distress, with hypoxemia and radiographic findings of diffuse pulmonary interstitial infiltrates, the center where the patient was transplanted should be contacted so that appropriate management can be discussed. Frequently, the approach will involve an open lung biopsy in order to obtain sufficient tissue to establish a reliable diagnosis. The diagnostic yield with transbronchial biopsies is often insufficient.

The attitude towards a return to normal activities will vary from patient to patient even in the absence of any significant medical problems. In general, patients should be encouraged to quickly expand their activities, and to keep physically and mentally active. Nevertheless, caution is indicated and a patient should not return to work or to school for at least 6 or possibly 9 months following transplantation. Again, most patients will easily comply with this since they often seem to lack the energy necessary to carry a full work load. It will also take some time for the patient to redevelop a normal appetite and enjoy food, which will allow him to consume the amount of calories necessary for normal performance. Food inake often increases with the gradual return of salivary secretion, and a recovery of smell and taste sensation after radiochemotherapy.

There should be little concern about household pets, plants, or working in the garden. However, caution is recommended in any contact with barnyard animals (because of fungal diseases and parasites), and swimming in public or private pools should be avoided because of the high frequency of heavy contamination with potentially pathogenic organisms. In any event, whenever outside for work or leisure, patients should use sun blocking creams to prevent actinic activation or reactivation of chronic GVHD (see below). Patients may resume normal sexual activity but constraint in the number of sexual partners is recommended.

Hematologic Function. Engraftment of donor marrow usually occurs within 2–3 weeks of transplantation, and granulocyte counts of $1 \times 10^9/l$ or greater are reached within one month of transplantation. Consequently, the patient no longer requires antibiotic coverage other than trimethoprim/sulfamethoxazole which is given 2 days/week for long term prophylaxis. Similarly, most patients become independent of platelet transfusions within 4–6 weeks of transplantation. It is quite rare that platelet transfusions are required beyond day 100, i.e. at the time the patient is usually returned to the care of the referring physician. In patients who receive cyclosporine as GVHD prophylaxis, a reticulocytopenic anemia possibly related to cyclosporine has been described. Since most patients receive cyclosporine for 6–12 months after transplantation, it may be necessary to support patients temporarily with transfusions of packed red blood cells. If transfusions are required they should be irradiated, at least during the first 6 months after transplantation, with approximately 2,000 rad in vitro to prevent the occurrence of transfusion-induced GVHD.

Another problem is marrow graft rejection. In contrast to transplantation of solid organs such as kidney or liver, where acute or chronic rejection are frequent problems, rejection is a rather infrequent event in bone marrow transplantation. If rejection is to occur, it usually does so during the early post grafting period. This problem is discussed in detail elsewhere (IV.3.).

Any change in hematological parameters should be investigated, not only from the point of view of graft failure, but also in regards to the possibility of recurrence of an underlying malignancy. However, a fall in leukocytes or platelets in peripheral blood might be due to other reasons including viral infections, progression of chronic GVHD, or myelosuppression by treatment for chronic GVHD with azathioprine. In any event, if changes occur a work-up including bone marrow aspiration and possibly biopsy should be obtained. If recurrent leukemia is suspected, it is helpful to have available bone marrow slides obtained at the time the patient's original diagnosis was established. Furthermore, if a marrow aspirate is obtained, samples should also be secured for cytogenetic analysis, particularly in patients in whom the donor was of different sex or when the original leukemia had an identifiable chromosomal marker. If there was no sex difference a sample to be analyzed for restriction fragment length polymorphism to determine donor or host origin should be obtained. In more than 95% of cases the recurrence of leukemia will be of the original host type. In the remaining cases, however, either a new leukemia in host-derived cells or a leukemia occurring in donor cells either of the same phenotype or a phenotype different from the original leukemia may be observed. Although most recurrences of leukemia following marrow transplantation will occur within 1–2 years of transplantation, late recurrences up to 6 years following transplantation have been observed. It is, in any case of recurrence, advisable and helpful to notify the center at which the patient was transplanted.

There are numerous other potential complications following marrow transplantation. The most important ones include chronic GVHD, ocular complications other than those associated with GVHD, problems with growth, development and fertility, pulmonary complications, and secondary malignancies, which are all discussed separately in the following chapters.

Since in many respects marrow transplantation is still an experimental procedure, the request by most transplant centers to have the patient return for a thorough re-evaluation, approximately one year after transplantation appears to be very appropriate. Since new problems are constantly being recognized and more importantly new methods of treatment are being established, optimum treatment can probably be provided only by an experienced team (see below).

References

Deeg HJ, Storb R, Thomas ED (1984) Bone marrow transplantation: A review of delayed complications. Br J Haematol 57: 185

Nicholls MD, Atkinson K, Biggs JC, Concannon AJ, Dodds AJ (1984) Late onset pyridoxine-responsive sideroblastic anaemia after allogeneic bone marrow transplantation. Br J Haematol 56: 153

Smith CI, Aarli JA, Biberfeld P, Bolme P, Christensson B, Gahrton G, Hammarstrom L, Lefvert AK, Lonnqvist B, Matell G, Pirskanen R, Ringden O, Svanborg E (1983) Myasthenia gravis after bone-marrow transplantation – Evidence for a donor origin. New Eng J Med 309: 1565

Spruce W, Forman S, McMillan R, Farbstein M, Turner M, Blume KG (1983) Idiopathic thrombocytopenic purpura following bone marrow transplantation. Acta Hematologica 69: 47

Sullivan KM, Deeg HJ, Sanders JE, Shulman HM, Witherspoon RP, Doney K, Appelbaum FR, Schubert MM, Stewart P, Springmeyer S, McDonald GB, Storb R, Thomas ED (1984) Late complications after marrow transplantation. Seminars in Hematol 21: 53

2. Chronic Graft-Versus-Host Disease

Chronic GVHD develops typically more than three months post transplant, and differs from acute GVHD in its distribution of target organs and clinical presentation. Although generally assumed, it has not been conclusively proven, that acute and chronic GVHD have the same immunopathogenesis: namely, the proliferation of mature donor T-cells in response to histocompatibility alloantigens of the host. In long term stable survivors without chronic GVHD this alloimmunity is apparently blocked by specific suppressor cells which usually are not found in patients with chronic GVHD. It has also been postulated that the establishment of tolerance requires a functioning thymus. Since thymus function can be destroyed by acute GVHD, the lack of thymus function may hamper the development of specific suppressor cells capable of mediating stable graft-host-tolerance. The donor-host directed alloagression may be only an initial event leading to autoimmune symptoms, impaired immune reconstitution and infections.

Clinical Manifestations of Chronic GVHD

Most patients developing chronic GVHD will have had preceding acute GVHD. Symptoms can develop either as a progressive extension of acute GVHD or following a quiescent period after resolution of acute GVHD. In addition, about 20–30% of patients will have de novo late onset GVHD without evidence of

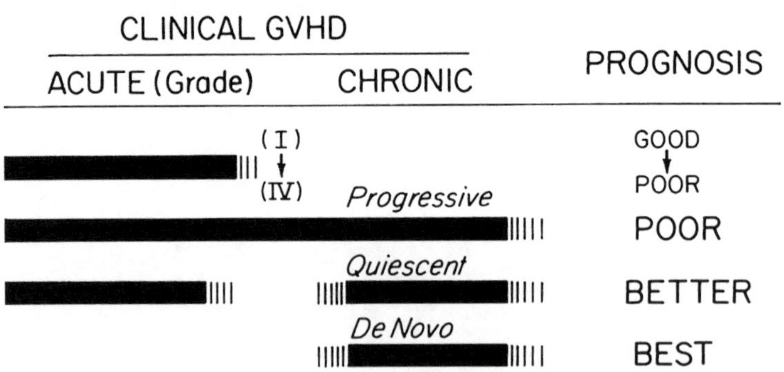

Fig. 8. Presentation of chronic GVHD relative to acute GVHD, as progressive, quiescent or de novo form

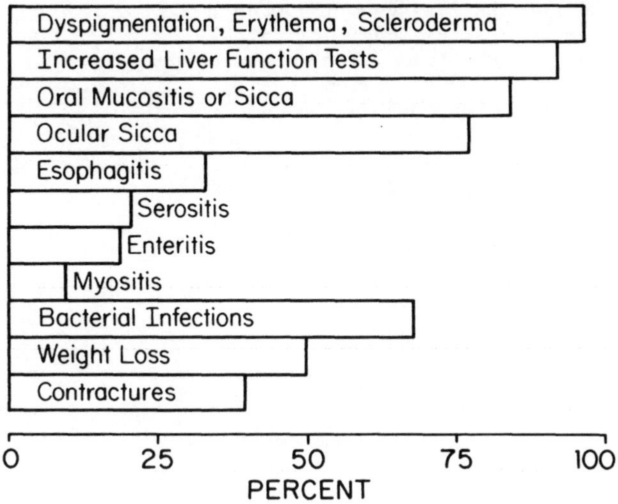

Fig. 9. Incidence of clinical manifestations in patients with extensive chronic GVHD. (Reprinted with permission from H. J. Deeg et al, Bone Marrow Transplantation: A Review of Delayed Complications, Br. J. Haematol. (1984) 57:185)

prior acute GVHD. Studies have shown that mortality is highest in those patients who have the progressive type onset chronic GVHD (Fig. 8).

The spectrum of clinical symptoms in patients with chronic GVHD resembles several known collagen vascular diseases such as scleroderma, systemic lupus erythematosus, lichen planus, Sjögren's syndrome, rheumatoid arthritis and primary biliary cirrhosis (Fig. 9). In contrast to several of these disorders, renal and CNS involvement is rarely seen in chronic GVHD. According to the extent of organ involvement, a clinicopathological classification has been developed which allows the discrimination between *"limited"* and *"extended"* chronic GVHD (Table 25). Except for chronic GVHD limited to the skin, it is unusual to have GVHD isolated to a single site.

Table 25. Clinicopathological Classification of Chronic Graft-Versus-Host Disease

Limited chronic graft-versus-host disease:
Either or Both:
* Localized skin involvement
* Hepatic dysfunction (due to chronic GVHD)

Extensive chronic graft-versus-host disease:
Either:
* Generalized skin involvement;

or
* Localized skin involvement or hepatic dysfunction due to chronic GVHD or both plus:
  - Liver histology showing chronic aggressive hepatitis, bridging necrosis, or cirrhosis: or
  - Involvement of eye (Schirmer's test with less than 5 mm wetting); or
  - Involvement of minor salivary glands or oral mucosa demonstrated on labial biopsy; or
  - Involvement of any other target organ

Adopted from Shulman and colleagues

Table 26. Skin Manifestations of Chronic GVHD

Early:	* Erythema with macules and plaques * Desquamation * Dyspigmentation * Vitiligo * Leukoderma * Lichen planus-like lesions * Nail abnormalities * Alopecia
Late:	* Induration * Contractures * Atrophy * Poikiloderma

Skin

Involvement of the skin by chronic GVHD occurs in more than 95% of patients. Early symptoms may include dryness, itching and loss of sweating while late symptoms are those of tightness and contracture. Raynaud's phenomenon is not common. Nail abnormalities, patchy alopecia, dyspigmentation and mucous membrane abnormalities are frequent (Table 26).

The onset of skin symptoms usually is more gradual, and preferentially occurs in sun exposed areas. However, an explosive onset of erythema and desquamation may occur after solar activation. Sometimes lichen planus-like lesions can herald a flare of skin GVHD. In some cases chronic GVHD of the skin can evolve, with an intense inflammatory phase with edematous areas and desquamation after minimal trauma. Skin lesions can occasionally be associated with dermal fields of total lymphoid irradiation and localized areas of cutaneous measles exanthema. Inadequately treated patients develop progressively indurated skin which is fixed to the underlying fascia. Clinically the picture resembles scleroderma with atrophic epidermis, thickened dermis and poikiloderma. A brown coloured patchy hyperpigmentation, joint contractures and skin ulcerations may complete the picture (Fig. 10).

Histopathologically, two major types of skin GVHD can be distinguished: the *generalized* type which is characterized by early epidermal hypertrophy and hyperkeratosis, clusters of eosinophilic bodies, and an increasing thickening of the basement membrane and the papillary dermis. Immunoglobulin (IgM) and complement deposits can be found at the dermal-epidermal junctions of cutaneous lesions. In the *localized* type, lichenoid reactions with eosinophilic bodies are rarely seen. Instead, dense focal dermal fibrosis and epidermal atrophy occur without any significant inflammation.

Mouth

Like skin involvement, involvement of the mouth is seen in a large proportion (80%) of patients with extensive chronic GVHD. The most frequent symptoms

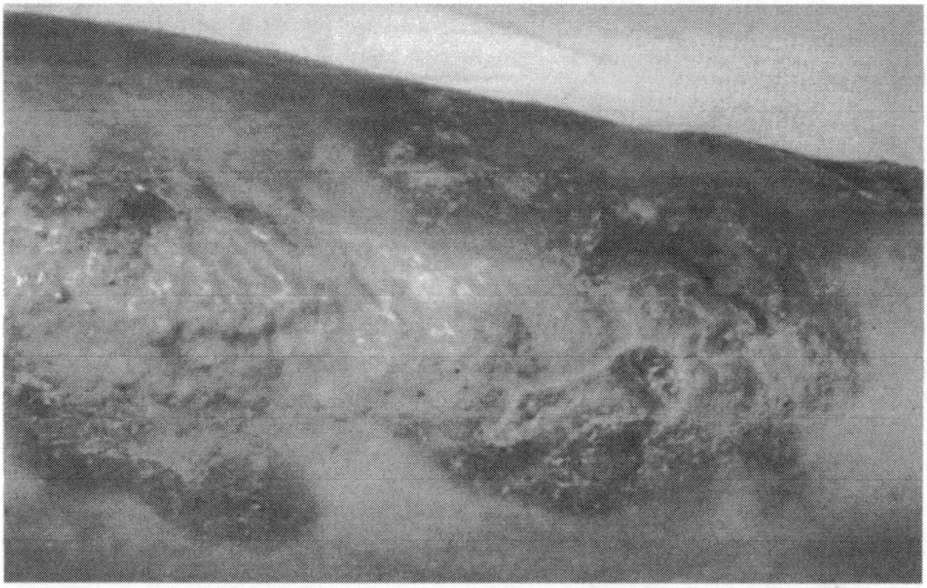

Fig. 10. Chronic GVHD of the skin after protracted course, with atrophy of the epidermis, induration of the dermis and ulcerations (sclerodermalike changes)

are pain, particularly with hot and warm foods, and dryness of the mucous membranes. Lichen planus-like lesions of the buccal and labial mucosa are common (Fig. 11) and can easily be misdiagnosed as oral candidiasis. Xerostomia may facilitate development of dental caries, periodontitis and atrophy of the filiform papillae. Histopathological changes include atrophy, necrosis of squamous cells and mononuclear cell infiltration characteristic of a lichenoid reaction. Salivary glands may show a lymphoplasmacytic cell infiltration around the ducts, ultimately leading to fibrosis of the gland.

Eyes

Occular involvement is observed in up to 80% of patients with extensive chronic GVHD. Most of the symptoms develop secondary to insufficient tear production as part of the sicca syndrome of chronic GVHD, which may cause pain, burning and photophobia. Occular sicca can also lead to keratitis and scarring. Histologic review reveals tarsal and conjunctival inflammation along with lacrimal gland fibrosis. Although less frequent, the uvea can also be involved by chronic GVHD: iritis, iridocyclitis and choroiditis can occur, and reflect the "autoimmune" character of chronic GVHD. To assess the extent of lacrimal insufficiency, a Schirmer's test is recommended. Pathological changes of the cornea (keratitis sicca) need evaluation by fluorescein biomicroscopy. Patients with "dry eyes" should

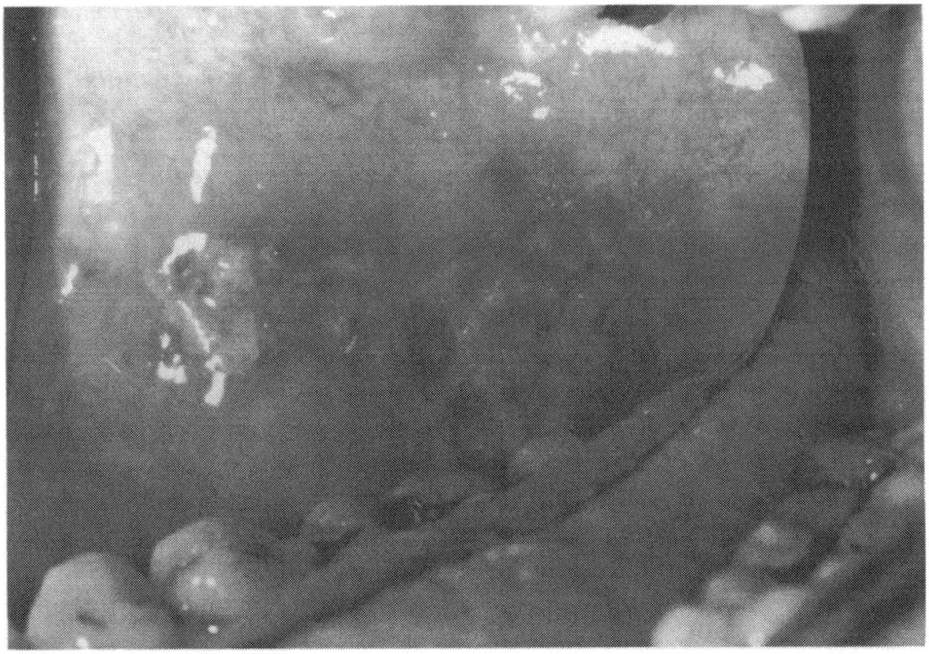

Fig. 11. Chronic GVHD of the oral mucosa, showing typical lichen planus-like changes. There is also neovascularization best visible in the upper part of the picture

use artificial tears to prevent progressive corneal erosion, perforation of scarring. When assessing eye involvement by chronic GVHD it should be remembered that long-term use of corticosteroids and total body irradiation can cause ocular problems, in particular cataract formation (see V.4). A sicca syndrome can also involve the mouth, the genital tract, in particular the vagina, and the mucosa of the tracheobronchial tree.

Gastrointestinal Tract

Esophagus

In contrast to acute GVHD, intestinal involvement by chronic GVHD is less common, and pathologic changes are most often seen in the esophagus. It can present as dysphagia, pain, swelling or retrosternal pain. "Web formation" associated with mucosal desquamation, strictures and partial occlusion along with functional abnormalities can be diagnosed by barium esophagogram, and are localized mainly in the upper esophagus (Fig. 12). Endoscopy may reveal epithelial peeling or desquamation. Manometric studies have shown a spectrum of motility disorders ranging from aperistalsis to high amplitude contraction. In

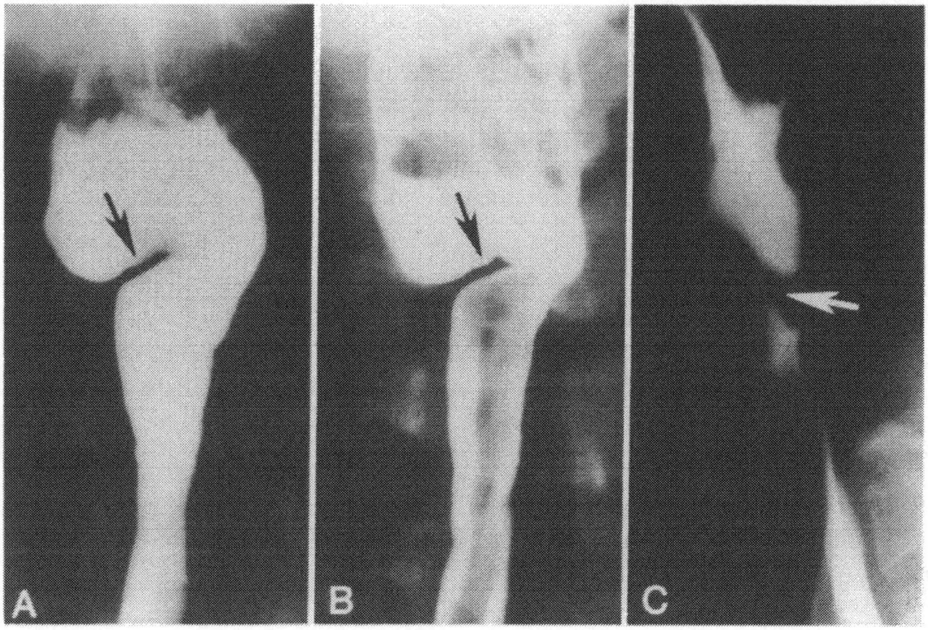

Fig. 12. Chronic GVHD of the esophagus. Radiograph of a barium swallow in an inadequately treated patient showing web formation, and partial occlusion. (Reproduced with permission from G. B. McDonald et al, "Radiographic features of esophageal involvement in chronic graft-vs-host disease", Am. J. Roentgenology 142:501, 1984)

contrast to scleroderma, esophageal muscle fibrosis is not characteristic of chronic GVHD. Histopathological alterations may include mononuclear cell inflammation, necrosis of squamous cells and submucosal fibrosis. Problems arise when the esophageal involvement causes symptoms such as dysphagia which may lead to poor caloric intake and weight loss. Esophageal obstruction can also cause aspiration and subsequent recurrent pulmonary disease. In order to prevent irreversible changes, it is important to recognize chronic GVHD of the esophagus early in the course and initiate appropriate immunosuppressive treatment.

Liver

About 90% of all patients with chronic GVHD also have various degrees of chronic liver disease. If it is associated with skin manifestations only, ("limited chronic GVHD") the outcome is usually more favorable than in patients with extensive chronic GVHD. Pathology and clinical picture of this complication are described in more detail in IV.6.

Gut

In contrast to acute GVHD, stomach and gut are rarely affected by chronic GVHD. In a screening program conducted in Seattle, only a few patients showed signs of chronic GVHD of the gut. Patients may have some diarrhea, crampy abdominal pain or both. Malabsorption can occur mostly related to fibrotic changes in the lamina propria, submucosa and mucosa.

Vagina

Extensive chronic GVHD may involve inflammation, sicca, adhesion and stenosis of the vagina. If chronic GVHD is not active, factors such as sequelae of total body irradiation and atrophy due to a lack of use should be considered. If atrophy is the most likely cause, dilators and estrogen creams are recommended. Systemic cyclic estrogen and progesterone combinations are also useful in preventing vaginal sclerosis. If chronic GVHD is suspected to significantly contribute to these vaginal problems, systemic immunosuppressive treatment is necessary. In some cases surgical intervention may be required.

Serosal Involvement

Some degree of serosal involvement is encountered in about 20% of patients with extensive chronic GVHD. Symptoms are secondary to pericardial, pleural and synovial effusions.

Lung

Obstructive lung disease has been increasingly recognized as a late manifestation of chronic GVHD. About 5–10% of long-term survivors with chronic GVHD may ultimately develop this type of complication which can be very resistant to treatment. Its clinical features are described in more detail in V.3.

Myasthenia Gravis

This naturally occuring disease is characterized by autoantibodies against the acetylcholine receptor. Recently a few patients with chronic GVHD have been described as meeting the diagnostic criteria for myasthenia gravis, such as the distribution of muscular weakness, response to edrophonium, repetitive nerve stimulation and antibodies against the acetylcholine receptor. Symptoms appeared late after transplant as corticosteroid therapy was being tapered. It is not clear at the moment which patients with chronic GVHD are at risk of developing myasthenia gravis. This manifestation of the disease is suspected to be related to immune dysregulation and donor-host alloreactivity. Other rare neuromuscular abnormalities in chronic GVHD may include *polymyositis* and *peripheral neuropathy*.

Autoimmune Problems

The clinical manifestations of chronic GVHD resemble those of some spontaneous autoimmune diseases. However, the autoantibody profile is significantly different in both disease entities. Antinuclear antibodies can be found in up to 80% of patients after marrow transplantation without any difference between patients with or without chronic GVHD. Antibodies against antinuclear antigen (native DNA and nuclear antigen) are usually negative. Occasionally antibodies against mitochondria, epidermal cells and smooth muscle cells are found without any clear correlation to the clinical picture. Some patients with GVHD may develop antiplatelet antibodies and autoimmune thrombocytopenia.

Immunodeficiency

Patients with chronic GVHD have delayed immune recovery and remain immunodeficient usually as long as the disease is active. Both B and T-cells can be quantitatively and qualitatively altered. Specifically, the percentage of suppressor cells remains increased along with a decreased number of helper cells. Since these helper cells usually produce a variety of lymphokines numerous T and B-cell functions are affected in a negative sense. In B-cells, the response to neo-antigens is delayed along with the ability of B-cells to switch from IgM production to IgG production in secondary responses.

In addition, patients with chronic GVHD often have a deficiency of intestinal secretory immunity and a reduced level of salivary IgA, particularly if the patient has GVHD related sialadenitis. This secretory IgA deficiency may contribute to the frequent sinobronchial infections observed in patients with chronic GVHD. In addition to disorders in the specific immune response, functions involving the nonspecific immune system are also defective such as granulocyte chemotaxis and opsonin activity of monocytes.

The pathogenesis of the delayed recovery of immune function in patients with chronic GVHD has not yet been sufficiently delineated. Some studies suggest that the normal maturation of T-cells is interrupted by specific blockages at one or more levels after grafting. Since the thymus plays a central role in educating lymphoid cells and is usually destroyed by acute GVHD and the preparative regimen, this lack of thymic education might contribute to the immunodeficiency in patients with chronic GVHD.

Infectious Complications in Patients with Chronic GVHD

Except for varizella zoster, the incidence of infections in long-term stable patients without chronic GVHD is not higher than in normal healthy people. However, the immunological disorders seen in patients with chronic GVHD predispose them to late infections, mostly with encapsulated bacteria.

Interstitial pneumonia developing later than day 100 after marrow transplantation occurs almost exclusively in patients with chronic GVHD.

There is still some uncertainty as to the best method of infection prophylaxis in these patients. Most patients will receive trimethoprim-sulfamethoxazole daily or at least twice weekly to protect them from infections with both pneumocystis carinii and gram positive organisms. If for some reason this drug cannot be given, penicillin is recommended instead. At some centers, ongoing studies are trying to answer the question of whether or not regular intravenous gammaglobulin application can effectively prevent infections in these patients.

Graft Versus Leukemia Effect

In 1956, Barnes observed that a transplanted marrow graft can destroy residual leukemic cells in lethally irradiated mice. This graft versus leukemia effect could also be shown in patients who develop acute GVHD, and is further supported by the observation that identical twins receiving a transplant for AML in first remission have a two-fold increase in relapse rate when compared to allogeneic recipients with the same disease. It is likely that chronic GVHD, particularly the de novo onset type, also has some antileukemic effect that may lead to improved long-term survival due to a decreased relapse rate. One study in children with ALL in relapse treated with HLA-identical transplant showed that there were no long-term survivors in the group of patients without acute or chronic GVHD, due to recurrent leukemia.

Diagnosis and Grading of Chronic GVHD

The diagnosis of chronic GVHD is based on clinical and histopathological criteria, and the clinician needs the pathologist to assess the response to treatment. A punch biopsy should be obtained from the involved skin. Even in the absence of a skin rash, a biopsy from the sun-exposed forearm can show diagnostic changes. Histopathological criteria for active skin disease include:
basal vascular degeneration,
eosinophilic body formation,
lymphoplasmocytic cell infiltration.

In addition, an oral biopsy approximately 5 mm long and 3 mm deep, from the inner lower lip should be obtained to establish and stage the activity of chronic GVHD. Other sites that may need histological confirmation are liver, esophagus, lung and muscle. Table 27 summarizes diagnostic procedures recommended to establish the diagnosis of limited or extensive clinical chronic GVHD. The severity of chronic GVHD and its impact on the patient is best graded by Karnofsky performance status (Table 28).

Table 27. Diagnostic Procedures to Assess Activity and Organ Involvement of Chronic GVHD

Screening Study	*Abnormality*
In all patients:	
Skin biopsy from forearm	Eosinophilic bodies, basal vacuoles
Oral/lip biopsy	Mucositis, sialadenitis
Schirmer's test	$\leq$ 5 mm wetting
Slit lamp examination	Corneal stippling
Liver function tests	Elevated
Pulmonary function tests	Forced midexpiratory flow decreased, FEV/FVC decreased
Recommended if symptoms are present:	
Upper GI endoscopy with biopsy	"Web" formation, strictures
Barium swallow (x-ray)	Desquamative esophagitis
Lower GI endoscopy with biopsy	Degeneration of glands, fibrosis in lamina propria, submucosa and serosa
Malabsorption tests	Stool fat increased

Table 28. Karnofsky Score

Karnofsky *Score (%)*	*Description*
100	Normal, no complaints; no evidence of disease.
90	Able to carry on normal activity; minor signs or symptoms of disease.
80	Normal activity with effort; some signs or symptoms of disease.
70	Cares for self and is well but unable to work. Requires infrequent outpatient follow-up and sees M.D. only once a week.
60	Requires occasional assistance but is able to care for most needs. Visits M.D. 2–3 times a week.
50	Requires considerable assistance and frequent medical care. Daily or alternate day M.D. visits are necessary.
40	Disabled and requires special care. If outpatient, requires special M.D./R.N. care; if inpatient, requires little active care (up, out of bed and in good condition).
30	Severely disabled and hospitalization is indicated although death is not imminent. Clinical condition is fair.
25	Hospitalization is mandated. Condition is fair to poor, but stable.
20	Active supporting treatment in hospital required. Condition is poor and unstable.
15	Active intensive care is continually required. Condition is critical.
10	Patient is moribund with a fatal process rapidly progressing. Condition is thought to be hypercritical.
5	Patient is moribund. Condition is terminal and irreversible. ("No code" status).
0	Patient is dead.

Predictive Factors

Factors which have been shown to be associated with an increased incidence of chronic GVHD include:

- Increasing age of the recipient
- Preceeding acute GVHD
- Infusion of non-irradiated donor buffy-coat cells after transplantation for aplastic anemia
- Second marrow infusion for poor graft function
- Non HLA identical transplants

In a recent study, 19% of long-term survivors with previous Grades 0–I acute GVHD developed chronic GVHD compared to 57% of survivors with Grades II–IV acute GVHD. Most centers assess the activity of chronic GVHD based on studies (Table 29) around 3 months post transplant ("day 100 workup"), and decide whether or not prolonged immunosuppressive treatment is required. In particular a positive skin or oral biopsy has a high predictive value: of those patients in whom this is the only sign of chronic GVHD (subclinical chronic GVHD), about 70% will develop overt active disease months later.

Patients requiring a second marrow infusion for poor graft function also have an increased incidence of chronic GVHD.

Prognostic Factors

The prognosis in patients who have limited disease is usually very good but is less favorable in those with untreated extensive chronic GVHD. In addition, the type of onset of chronic GVHD has some prognostic meaning; chronic GVHD which progresses from unresolved acute GVHD, has an unfavorable prognosis. In contrast, patients with de novo onset chronic GVHD (no preceding acute GVHD) have the best prognosis, and those with quiescent onset, which arises after complete resolution of acute GVHD, have an intermediate prognosis. Furthermore, it is known that patients with extensive chronic GVHD and persistent thrombocytopenia ($<100 \times 10^9$/L) have an increased mortality. The pathogenesis of thrombocytopenia is largely unknown, but is assumed to be related to the immunoregulatory abnormalities in GVHD.

Prophylaxis of Chronic GVHD

Since *acute* GVHD represents a risk factor for the development of subsequent chronic GVHD, attempts to prevent chronic GVHD are aimed at reducing incidence and severity of acute GVHD. *Methotrexate* and *cyclosporine* either alone or in combination are administered starting shortly before and shortly after marrow infusion and at regular intervals thereafter to prevent acute GVHD. Further prophylactic modalities include T-cell depletion of the donor marrow by various methods or total lymphoid irradiation as part of the conditioning regimen (IV.2). Prolonged administration of corticosteroids (from the time of engraftment until 18 months post grafting) was found to be successful in preventing chronic GVHD at one center but was not confirmed by others. In patients with severe aplastic anemia some investigators have omitted the infusion of viable donor buffy coat cells, thus decreasing the probability of chronic GVHD. However, to achieve engraftment it was necessary to incorporate total body or total lymphoid irradiation into the conditioning regimen. Since, conceivably, irradiation will result in delayed effects other than GVHD in patients with otherwise non-malignant diseases, this approach should be used cautiously.

Treatment of Extensive Chronic GVHD

Patients who have limited chronic GVHD (Table 26) are usually not treated and, instead, are monitored closely to observe any progression of the disease. The natural course of *extensive* chronic GVHD is unfavorable and less than 20% of untreated patients become longterm survivors free of disability. There are a few anecdotal reports on untreated patients whose chronic GVHD "burnt-out" 5–10 years post BMT. However, these patients are severely disabled from contractures, runting and blindness. Treatment has to be instituted early in the course of chronic GVHD, since late therapy cannot influence the unfavorable course of the disease. In the past steroids alone or in combination with azathioprine and cyclophosphamide with procarbazine have been used. The rate of disability-free survival in patients treated with steroids plus azathioprine was around 75% in initial studies from Seattle. This combination was less favorable for patients who had failed initial prednisone treatment than for those treated initially with the combination.

Patients who have extensive chronic GVHD along with persistent thrombocytopenia (platelets less thann 100×10^9/L) or those who have failed initial therapy of chronic GVHD belong to a "high risk" group and require more intensive treatment for a longer period of time. The combination of prednisone and cyclosporine is, at the moment, the most efficacious combination. The dosage schedule of the two drugs differs somewhat from center to center. The Seattle group introduced an alternate-day regimen giving 1 mg/kg/day prednisone on day A, and cyclosporine 6 mg/kg every 12 hours on day B. Modifications of this regimen are being explored: the simultaneous administration of prednisone and cyclosporine for a couple of weeks as induction therapy and the subsequent administration of cyclosporine only as maintenance for a total of 9–12 months. Other centers prefer to give cyclosporine as a single treatment and add corticosteroids when the disease flares. Some cases with drug resistant chronic GVHD of the mouth or skin may benefit from a combination of psoralen and ultraviolet irradiation (PUVA). GVHD confined to the mouth can be treated with some success by mouth rinsing with corticosteroids (decadron 0.25%). More recently, thalidomide has shown some effects in otherwise treatment resistant chronic GVHD.

Usually activity of chronic GVHD is assessed at 1 year with the same studies performed on day 100 post transplant. About 25% of all patients may have a flare of GVHD activity within the first 6 months after discontinuation of the immunosuppressive treatment. Depending on severity, it may be necessary to resume treatment. However, if the patient is stable and off immunosuppressive therapy for more than 6 months, permanent tolerance is most likely and a late "relapse" is rarely seen.

Supportive Care

These measures are primarily aimed at preventing recurrent infection and disability. They include prophylactic antibiotics, oral hygiene, artificial saliva and tears, nutritional support and sun-blocking creams (grade $\geq$ 15). To prevent vaginal stenosis, topical estrogen creams as well as systemic estrogen/progesterone combinations are recommended. To prevent esophageal disease, antacids, ranitidine and elevation of the head of the bed may be employed.

References

Atkinson K, Incefy GS, Storb R, Sullivan KM, Iwata T, Dardene M, Ochs HD, Good RA, Thomas ED (1982) Low serum thymic hormone levels in patients with chronic graft-versus-host disease. Blood 59: 1073

Atkinson K, Weller P, Ryman W, Biggs J (1986) PUVA therapy for drug-resistant graft-versus-host disease. Bone Marrow Transplantat 1: 227

Corson SL, Sullivan K, Batzer F, August C, Storb R, Thomas ED (1982) Gynecologic manifestations of chronic graft-versus-host disease. Obstet Gynecol 60: 488

Franklin RM, Kenyon KR, Tutschka PJ, Saral R, Green WR, Santos G (1983) Occular manifestations of graft versus host disease. Ophthalmology 90: 4

Gratwohl AA, Moutsopoulos HM, Chused TM, Akizuki M, Wolf RO, Sweet JB, Deisseroth AB (1977) Sjögren-type syndrome after allogeneic bone-marrow transplantation. Ann Int Med 87: 703

Klingemann H-G, Lum LG, Storb R (1987) Phenotypical and functional studies on a subtype of suppressor cells ($CD8^+/CD11^+$) in patients after bone marrow transplantation. Transplantation 44: 381

Lum LG (1987) The kinetics of immune reconstitution after human marrow transplantation. Blood 69: 369

McDonald GB, Sullivan K, Plumley TF (1984) Radiographic features of esophageal involvement in chronic graft-vs-host disease. Am J Radiol 142: 501

Ringden O, Paulin T, Lönnqvist B, Nilsson B (1985) An analysis of factors predisposing to chronic graft-versus-host disease. Exp Hematol 13: 1062

Rouquette-Gally AM, Boyeldieu D, Gluckman E, Abuaf N, Combrisson A (1987) Autoimmunity in 28 patients after allogeneic bone marrow transplantation: comparison with Sjögren syndrome and scleroderma. Br J Haematol 66: 45

Sale GE, Shulmann HM, Schubert MM, Sullivan KM, Kopecky KJ, Hackman RC, Morton TH, Storb R, Thomas ED (1981) Oral and ophthalmic pathology of graft versus host disease in man: predictive value of the lip biopsy. Hum Pathol 12: 1022

Saurat JH, Gluckman E, Bussel A, Didierjean L, Puissant A (1975) The lichen planus-like eruption after bone marrow transplantation. Br J Dermatol 92: 675

Schubert HM, Sullivan KM, Morton TH, Izutsu KT, Peterson DE, Flournoy N, Truelove EL, Sale GE, Buckner CD, Storb R, Thomas ED (1984) Oral manifestation of chronic graft versus host disease. Ann Intern Med 144: 1591

Shulman HM, Sullivan KM, Weiden PL et al. (1980) Chronic graft-versus-host syndrome in man. Am J Med 69: 204

Sullivan KM, Shulman HM, Storb R, Weiden PL, Witherspoon RP, McDonald GB, Schubert MM, Atkinson K, Thomas ED (1981) Chronic graft-versus-host disease in 52 patients: adverse natural course and successful treatment with combination immunosuppression. Blood 57: 267

Sullivan KM (1986) Acute and chronic graft-versus-host disease in man. Int J Cell Clon 4: 42

Weiden PL, Sullivan KM, Flournoy N et al. (1981) Antileukemic effect of chronic graft versus host disease. Contributions to improved survival after allogeneic marrow transplantation. N Eng J Med 304: 1529

3. Pulmonary Problems

Acute pulmonary toxicity early after transplantation is mainly related to high dose chemoradiotherapy and manifests itself as interstitial pneumonitis. However, there are also numerous infectious agents that can affect the lung early post-transplant.

The probability of infectious complications of the lung decreases with time after transplant. However, in recipients who develop chronic GVHD, pulmonary infections, even recurrent, can occur as a delayed problem. These infections are presumably related to a decrease in the mucociliary clearance mechanism, immunoregulatory defects, and the reduced production of secretory IgA. Acute pulmonary infections are described in more detail in IV.4 and IV.5.

In addition to infections caused by classic pathogens or viruses, a spectrum of other pulmonary complications can be encountered late after allogeneic bone marrow transplantation:

- Restrictive pulmonary disease
- Obstructive pulmonary disease
- Pulmonary vascular abnormalities

Restrictive Pulmonary Disease

Restrictive defects of ventilatory function are common in transplanted patients. Even in otherwise healthy long term survivors, sequential pulmonary function studies have shown a mean loss in total lung capacity of 0.81 litres, a decrease in vital capacity of 0.54 litres, and an impairment of diffusing capacity of 4.4 ml/min/mmHg at one year after bone marrow transplantation in up to 21% of patients. However, in this particular study, lung function improved again over the subsequent 3 to 4 years. The restrictive pulmonary changes are apparently not correlated with any particular type of conditioning regimen or the presence of chronic GVHD, although it is known that chemotherapy can cause interstitial pulmonary changes with subsequent fibrosis and restrictive losses in function. Patients with interstitial pneumonitis in the early post-transplant course tend to have greater restrictive changes subsequently than patients without preceding pneumonitis. Generally these restrictive pulmonary alterations are mild, do not produce severe symptoms and therefore, do not require therapeutic intervention. It is not clear, however, at the moment if and to what extent restrictive lung changes ultimately contribute to obstructive pulmonary alterations.

Obstructive Pulmonary Disease

Some patients develop obstructive pulmonary problems following marrow transplantation. About 10% of patients studied for four or more years after transplant had forced expiratory volumes less than 50% of predicted. The pathogenesis of obstructive airway disease after marrow transplantation is largely unknown. In some instances, obstructive lung disease might be a sequel of extensive restrictive changes in the small airways. Evidence is also accumulating that some cases may be related to chronic GVHD.

In general, one has to distinguish between the moderate obstruction after transplantation that can occur in patients who have received chemo- and radiotherapy, and obstructive lung disease due to lymphocytic bronchitis or bronchiolitis obliterans, which can be recognized histologically and frequently occurs in conjunction with chronic GVHD.

Lymphocytic Bronchitis is often associated with a non-productive cough, dyspnea, wheezing and sometimes bronchospasm. Histologically, small lymphocytes can be seen infiltrating the proximal bronchial mucosa, submucosa and muscularis, and there is an associated loss of ciliae. Mucosal necrosis and submucosal gland necrosis contribute to the loss of mucous ciliary clearance.

Most of these patients also have oral mucositis, esophagitis, sinusitis and oral and ocular sicca syndrome or other symptoms related to chronic GVHD. Another frequent finding is a decreased serum IgA level which may predispose to recurrent infections of smaller airways, ultimately leading to chronic obstructive lung disease. Moreover, repeated aspiration caused by esophageal abnormalities related to chronic GVHD may also contribute to the pathogenesis of obstructive lung disease. Similarly, sinusitis is a frequent problem after transplantation, and the aspiration of purulent sinus secretions may be causative in the development of chronic obstructive airway disease. Therefore, patients with signs of chronic pulmonary problems, such as dry cough, wheezing, and dyspnea on exertion, should undergo the following studies:
Pulmonary function tests,
Sinus and esophageal radiography,
Tests to exclude indolent infection,
Tests to evaluate the activity of chronic GVHD.

Early treatment of the underlying disorder may prevent the development of obstructive lung disease in these patients.

Bronchiolitis Obliterans. Progressive bronchiolitis obliterans has also been linked to chronic GVHD. Bronchiolitis obliterans affects about 10% of all patients who have active chronic GVHD, and its clinical course can vary from mild and slow progression to diffuse necrotising bronchiolitis of the small airways leading to death of the patient. Additional risk factor include HLA-nonidentical grafts and immunosuppressive therapy with methotrexate. Chest films may show hyperinflation of the lungs, and flattening of the diaphragm. Recurrent pneumothoraces have been reported. Pulmonary function tests can show a marked reduction in forced midexpiratory flow to between 10 and 20% of predicted values, and moderate to severe reduction in FEV_1/FVC*. These changes indicate airflow obstruction especially involving small airways. In contrast, the carbon monoxide transfer coefficient is normal in these patients suggesting good gas exchange in the lung tissue being ventilated.

Additional diagnostic procedures may be helpful in some cases and unrevealing in others. Pulmonary ventilation scan can show decreased activity patterns corresponding to areas of reduced perfusion. Delayed clearance of the radioisotope may also be noted. Histological changes can be nonspecific, sometimes showing obliteration of bronchiolar walls along with atelectatic areas. A similar disease entity has been described in association with connective tissue disorders including rheumatoid arthritis and Sjoegrens' syndrome. This is of interest since chronic GVHD has many other features resembling collagen vascular disorders.

Significant morbidity among patients with bronchiolitis obliterans is caused by recurrent respiratory tract infections, often due to Pseudomonas aeruginosa. The reasons for these infections may include:

- low levels of secretory IgA
- damage to submucosal glands
- reduced mucociliary activity related to the sicca syndrome
- general impairment of humoral and cellular immunity.

Bronchiolitis obliterans has been observed as early as three months after marrow transplantation. The majority of patients tend to develop it within two years after marrow grafting. In progressive cases treatment options are limited, and characteristically this disease does not respond very well to therapy with bronchodilators. Prompt treatment of infections as well as appropriate therapy of chronic GVHD seem to be of benefit in this disease. Some centers give a 14 day course of high dose steroids (10 mg/kg) to get the disease under control and then maintain control with established chronic GVHD treatment protocols such as the combination of cyclosporine/prednisone.

Pulmonary Vascular Events

Pulmonary thrombi/emboli have been found at autopsy in up to 50% of patients after allogeneic bone marrow transplantation. These emboli are usually scattered and demonstrated only in arterioles, capillaries and venules. Usually there are no signs of muscular hyperplasia or intimal thickening. It is difficult to assess whether these pulmonary emboli can contribute to any abnormalities in pulmonary function after marrow transplantation such as decrease in diffusing capacity. The etiology is not clear. It may be that the infusion of even filtered bone marrow can cause some thrombosis in pulmonary vessels.

* FEV_1 = Forced expiratory volume in 1 second/FVC = Forced vitaly capacity

References

Beschorner WE, Saral R, Hutchins GM, Tutschka PJ, Santos GW (1978) Lymphocytic bronchitis associated with graft-versus-host disease in recipients of bone marrow transplants. N Eng J Med 229: 1030

Clark JG, Schwartz DA, Flournoy N, Sullivan KM, Crawford SW, Thomas ED (1987) Risk factors for airflow obstruction in recipients of bone marrow transplants. Ann Intern Med 107: 648

Hamilton PJ, Pearson ADJ (1986) Bone Marrow transplantation and the lung. Thorax 41: 497

Kurzrock R, Zander A, Kanojia M, Vellekoop L, Spitzer G, Jagannath S, Schell S, Peters L, Dicke K (1984) Obstructive lung disease after allogeneic bone marrow transplantation. Transplantation 37: 156

Link H, Reinhard U, Blaurock M, Ostendorf P (1986) Lung function changes after allogeneic bone marrow transplantation. Thorax 41: 508

Ralph DD, Springmeyer AC, Sullivan VM, Hackman RC, Storb R, Thomas ED (1984) Rapidly progressive air-flow obstruction in marrow transplant recipients. Am Rev Respir Dis 129: 641

Springmeyer SC, Silvestri RC, Flournoy N et al (1984) Pulmonary function of marrow transplant patients. 1. Effects of marrow infection, acute graft versus host disease, and interstitial pneumonitis. Exp Hematol 12: 805

4. Endocrine Function, Growth, and Development

Radiochemotherapy affects not only the intended target cells and tissues, i.e. lymphohemopoietic cells and tumor cells, but the organism as a whole. The most important factor is irradiation. Adverse effects are fewer, less severe or shorter lasting in patients conditioned with chemotherapy alone.

Thyroid Function

Thyroid function abnormalities and thyroid neoplasms have been well documented in patients given irradiation to the head or neck. It would not be surprising, therefore, to find similar abnormalities after TBI. Since the number of patients studied is still quite limited, an exact figure for the incidence of thyroid dysfunction cannot be given. It is clear, however, from studies at several marrow transplant centers that asymptomatic compensated hypothyroidism, overt hypothyroidism, or hyperthyroxinemia occur in a substantial proportion of patients, possibly as many as 40–50%. Elevated TSH and decreased T4 levels were observed as early as one and as late as fifteen years after transplant. In the most comprehensive study to date, reported by Sanders et al., no significant correlation of thyroid function abnormalities with previous cranial irradiation, fractionated or single dose TBI, presence or absence of chronic GVHD, patient age or sex was found. Overall, it appears that the incidence of these abnormalities is substantially higher than in patients given only cranial irradiation. Since untreated compensated hypothyroidism has been suggested as an important factor in the development of neoplastic thyroid disease, it is advisable to treat these patients with thyroid supplementation, and re-evaluate them sequentially for many years following transplantation.

Adrenal Glands

Only limited data on adrenal gland dysfunction following transplantation are available. In a study by Sanders and colleagues, 24% of 78 patients examined from 1–8 years after transplant (while not on glucocorticoid treatment) had subnormal 11-desoxycortisol levels. None of these patients was symptomatic, and the percentage of patients developing abnormalities appeared to remain relatively constant with time after transplant. No significant correlation with any patient characteristic was found. Although this study did not differentiate between primary and secondary adrenal insufficiency, the finding of subnormal stimulated cortisol levels is similar to that reported in patients given central nervous system irradiation. Further studies are necessary to determine whether these patients are able to handle physiological stress in a normal fashion.

Growth

Growth hormone deficiency is observed after central nervous system irradiation. In the study by Sanders and colleagues children underwent a growth hormone stimulation test with L-dopa or insulin, and among 25 patients evaluated, 21 showed some degree of growth hormone deficiency. Among 18 patients who had not received previous cranial irradiation only 6 had partial growth hormone deficiency.

It is likely that growth hormone deficiency contributed to some extent to decreased growth rates after TBI. However, other factors are also thought to be involved. Both male and female pediatric patients given TBI showed suppressed growth velocity curves and lacked a growth spurt in early adolescence. Growth velocity was further dampened in patients who also suffered from chronic GvHD. This change in growth velocity did not appear to be dependent upon treatment of chronic GvHD with glucocorticoids. It was also of note, that no catch-up growth was observed after discontinuing treatment for chronic GvHD. Furthermore, the lag in age adjusted growth did not decrease with increasing time after transplantation. Growth impairment was more severe with single dose TBI than with fractionated TBI, and in patients given previous cranial irradiation than in those without prior cranial irradiation. These correlations were particularly evident in male patients. Furthermore, the younger the patient was at the time of irradiation and the higher the dose of TBI, the more severe was growth retardation. The fact that the type of TBI (single dose vs fractionated) did not affect growth until approximately three years following transplant suggests that fractionated TBI allows for some repair and recovery, albeit delayed, of epiphyseal, metaphyseal, and diaphyseal bone growth. For the majority of patients radiological bone age was within two years of the chronologic age. Only a small fraction of patients lagged behind more than 2 years, and half of those had chronic GVHD which generally had been treated with glucocorticoids.

The fact that children do not show growth acceleration after discontinuing treatment with glucocorticoids has led to speculation that somatomedin may be abnormal (due to impaired synthesis in the liver), and thus, may contribute to abnormal growth rates. It is also conceivable that abnormal sex hormone levels play a role in this multifactorial growth abnormality. It will furthermore, be of interest to determine whether children treated for GVHD without glucocorticoids, for example with cyclosporine, show improved linear growth rates.

Sexual Development

Pubertal development and gonadal function have been of great concern in pediatric transplant patients. Sanders et al. studied 35 girls and 63 boys, 1–13 years of age. The majority of children, who were prepubertal at the time of TBI, showed delayed development and slow progression of secondary sexual characteristics due to primary (hypergonadotropic) hypogonadism.

In girls the development of breast stage and public hair according to the criteria of Tanner and Whitehouse was delayed in virtually all instances. Six girls had delayed menarche. However, all seventeen girls who were past puberty at the time of transplantation remained amenorrheic with elevated LH and FSH levels, and decreased estradiol levels for at least 2 years following transplantation. Subsequently, with follow-up from 3–14 years, some of these women have shown recovery of ovarian function with hormonal levels returning toward normal. Among 4 who had spontaneous menses 3–5 years after transplantation, one became pregnant and had an elective abortion. In order to avoid symptoms of menopause, cyclic hormone supplementation should be offered.

Similarly, boys had delayed pubertal development of penis and pubic hair stage, as well as testicular volume. Many boys had normal LH levels associated with normal FSH and testosterone levels, and these showed higher developmental scores than those with abnormal levels. Overall, among the 25 boys tested, 10 had elevated LH levels and 23 had elevated FSH levels, but testosterone was normal in all of them. Semen analysis, available in 4 boys, showed azoospermia.

In patients conditioned with regimens not containing TBI there was only very mild derangement of growth and sexual development. Within months of transplantation vertical growth resumed and patients appeared to reach normal height. There was a mild delay in sexual development but no lasting impairment seemed to occur. Unless interferred with by severe chronic GVHD, development was normal.

Fertility

Although retardation of skeletal growth or the development of secondary sexual characteristics among adult patients may not be of concern, all other potential problems described for pediatric patients apply here as well.

Sanders and colleagues evaluated gonadal functions in 130 patients, 1–11 years after marrow transplantation. More than 90% of women conditioned with TBI and chemotherapy continued to show elevated levels of luteinizing hormone and follicle stimulating hormone, and were amenorrheic. Only 3 of 38 women (8%) menstruated following transplantation. Two patients became pregnant and both had abortions.

In women conditioned with chemotherapy alone, generally cyclophosphamide, the outcome was strongly dependent upon age at the time of transplantation. Whereas all patients less than 26 years of age had a return to normal levels of luteinizing hormone and follicle stimulating hormone as well as menstruation, about two thirds of women 26 years of age or older continued to show elevated levels of these hormones, and remained amenorrheic. Five women less than 26 years of age became pregnant. Of these, three delivered normal children and two had abortions.

Results were somewhat different in men. Among patients given TBI and chemotherapy more than 90% were azoospermic, and 70–80% had elevated follicle stimulating hormone levels. However, almost 90% of patients had normal luteinizing hormone levels, and frequently had normal plasma testosterone. One man with a return of sperm production fathered two normal children.

Among men conditioned with chemotherapy only, approximately two thirds had a return of sperm production and a normalization of follicle stimulating hormone, and all but one had normal luteinizing hormone levels. Four men conditioned with chemotherapy only fathered five normal children.

Thus, in the adult population, the impact of the conditioning regimen used for marrow transplantation is less severe than in the pediatric population, but certainly is significant in regards to gonadal function. In women with iatrogenic menopause, hormone supplementation to prevent secondary complications of menopause such as vaginitis is advisable.

References

Deeg HJ, Kennedy MS, Sanders JE, Thomas ED, Storb R (1983) Successful pregnancy after marrow transplantation for severe aplastic anemia and immunosuppression with cyclosporine. JAMA 240: 647

Sanders JE, Buckner CD, Leonard JM, Sullivan KM, Witherspoon RP, Deeg HJ, Storb RL, Thomas ED (1983) Late effects on gonadal function of cyclophosphamide, total-body irradiation, and marrow transplantation. Transplantation 36: 252

Sanders JE, Pritchard S, Mahoney P, Amos D, Buckner CD, Witherspoon RP, Deeg HJ, Doney KC, Sullivan KM, Appelbaum FR, Storb R, Thomas ED (1986) Growth and development following marrow transplantation for leukemia. Blood 68: 1129

Sklar CA, Kim TH, Ramsay NK (1982) Thyroid dysfunction among longterm survivors of bone marrow transplantation. Am J Med 73: 688

Sklar CA, Kim TH, Williamson JF, Ramsay NK (1983) Ovarian function after successful bone marrow transplantation in postmenarcheal females. Med Pediatr Oncol 11: 361

Tichelli A, Gratwohl A, Speck B, Osterwalder B, Nissen C, Lori A, Wursch A, Walther E, Roth J, Hunig R (1986) Nebenwirkungen der Ganzkörperbestrahlung im Rahmen der Knochenmarktransplantation: Prophylaxe und Therapie. Schweiz. med. Wschr. 116: 1560

5. Ocular Problems

During and following marrow transplantation the eye can be damaged in many ways. The conjunctivae can be affected by certain chemotherapeutic agents and by viruses, the lacrimal glands can be involved by chronic GVHD, and there can be retinal hemorrhage and choroiditis (see above). In addition, there can be longterm effects, mostly affecting the lens.

It is known that irradiation can damage the ocular lens and lead to cataracts. This has been shown in patients undergoing localized irradiation to fields including the eyes, and in survivors of the atomic bomb explosions in Japan. Thus, it was expected that patients given TBI in preparation for marrow transplantation would also develop cataracts. We reported a study on 277 patients followed for 1–12 years after transplant. These patients had been prepared either with chemotherapy alone, or with TBI in combination with chemotherapy, with TBI being given as a single exposure or fractionated. Single dose TBI consisted of 10 Gy, fractionated TBI ranged from 12–15 Gy given over several days. While approximately 80% of patients given single dose TBI developed cataracts over a course of 5–6 years following transplantation, only 20% of patients given fractionated TBI did so. The incidence with fractionated TBI was, in fact, identical to that observed with chemotherapy regimens only, and was thought to be related in part at least to concurrent treatment of these patients with glucocorticoids. All cataracts involved the posterior capsule of the lens. Furhter analysis showed that the risk of developing cataracts was highest about 3 years after transplant, and subsequently declined. It was also of note that patients developing cataracts after single dose TBI were more symptomatic than those developing cataracts with fractionated TBI or with chemotherapy only. At least 50% of patients who developed cataracts after single dose TBI required surgical intervention within 2–6 years following transplant, in contrast to only 20% of patients given fractionated TBI, and none of the patients given chemotherapy only. The risk for developing cataracts was somewhat higher in patients with acute lymphoblastic leukemia and with chronic myelogenous leukemia than in patients with acute myeloid leukemias. The reason for this was not clear. However, it is conceivable that factors such as the prior use of steroids, cranial irradiation, or busulfan might predispose to the development of cataracts following transplantation.

Cataracts after marrow transplantation can be treated as in any other patient if no chronic GVHD of the eyes exists. Therefore, the treatment would be implantation of intraocular lenses, or if for some reason this is not feasible, the use of contact lenses. In patients, who have chronic GVHD and suffer from sicca syndrome of the eyes, one may want to delay intervention and one certainly should avoid the use of contact lenses. In this setting, therefore, the only solution would be cataract glasses which is not very satisfactory. Every effort should be made to improve the patient's condition, such that a lens can be implanted into the eye.

Irradiation to the eyes has also been reported to cause retinopathy within 1–3 years following exposure. Findings included vascular occlusions, hemorrhages, microaneurysms, neovascularization, retinal detachments and optic atrophy. These patients had generally been given 4,000–5,000 cGy or even higher doses to the eye. Although certain "nonspecific" ocular changes including retinal, have been observed after TBI and marrow transplantation, the doses used (920–1,575 cGy) were in a range where radiation retinopathy would not be expected.

References

Deeg HJ, Flournoy N, Sullivan KM, Sheehan K, Buckner CD, Sanders JE, Storb R, Witherspoon RP, Thomas ED (1984) Cataracts after total body irradiation and marrow transplantation: A sparing effect of dose fractionation. Int J Radiation Oncology Biol Phys 10: 957

Franklin RM, Kenyon KR, Tutschka PJ, Saral R, Green WR, Santos GW (1983) Ocular manifestations of graft-vs-host disease. Ophthalmology 90: 4

Jack MK, Jack GM, Sale GE, Shulman HM, Sullivan KM (1983) Ocular manifestations of graft versus host disease. Arch Ophthamol 101: 1080

Wara WM, Irvine AR, Neger RE, Howes EL, Phillips TL (1979) Radiation retinopathy. Int J Radiation Oncology Biol Phys 5: 81

6. Secondary Malignancies

As marrow transplantation has been used more frequently and with greater success, the number of long-term survivors has grown steadily. Consequently, the probability of detecting long-term side effects of marrow transplantation has increased. As described above, patients are usually prepared for transplantation by the administration of high doses of immunosuppressive/cytotoxic agents and TBI given either alone or in combination. Following the transplant procedure, patients go through a period of profound immunoincompetence. In addition, most of them receive immunosuppressive drugs such as methotrexate, cyclosporine or, methylprednisolone, in an attempt to prevent or treat GVHD. Cytotoxic agents, ionizing irradiation, and the use of immunosuppressive drugs are known to be associated with an increased risk of developing malignancies. Malignant tumors have been observed in patients given immunosuppressive treatment after renal or cardiac transplantation. Furthermore, a high incidence of malignant lymphomas has been observed in F_1 hybrid mice given parental hemopoietic grafts. Consequently, there has been concern that patients given TBI and marrow grafts might also be at increased risk of developing secondary malignancies. Studies in dogs and rhesus monkeys given allogeneic or autologous marrow grafts have, indeed, shown an increased incidence of malignant tumors as compared to control animals.

Clinical results suggest that there are four types of malignancies that occur after marrow transplantation: firstly, the recurrence of leukemia, identical in lineage and phenotype to the original disease, but developing in donor derived cells; second, lymphoproliferative disorders differing from the original disease; third, solid tumors; and fourth, new leukemias (Table 29).

The occurrence of leukemia in donor cells was first reported in 1971. The pathogenesis is not clear although several hypotheses have been proposed. Conceivably, donor lymphoid cells might undergo transformation due to antigenic stimulation by host tissue as observed in mouse models of marrow transplantation. This appears less likely in man. If this were the case, one would expect similar events in all human patients undergoing marrow transplantation. However, so far secondary malignancies have been observed predominantly (although not exclusively) in patients whose initial disease was malignant, and who were conditioned with regimens including the use of TBI. Alternatively, the host milieu in which the original leukemia had arisen might predispose to abnormal lymphohemopoietic maturation and proliferation of donor derived cells. It has also

Table 29. Secondary Malignancies

- * Recurrence of leukemia in donor-derived cells
- * Lymphoproliferative disorders (donor > host origin)
  - EBV positive
  - EBV negative
- * Solid tumors (host origin)
  - Adenocarcinoma
  - Squamous cell carcinoma
  - Glioblastoma multiforme
  - Malignant melanoma
  - Sarcoma
- * Leukemia in host cells of lineage different from original disease

been suggested that normal cells might undergo fusion with residual host leukemia cells, and, following diploidization, give rise to new malignancies. Finally, an etiologic agent such as an oncogene or a virus present in host cells may be transferred (transfected) to donor cells. Initial reports suggested that recurrences in donor cells usually occurred very early after transplantation, but this has now been observed as late as six years after transplant. Preliminary analyses suggest that recurrences may be in donor derived cells in approximately 5% of the observed cases. With the application of molecular biology techniques such as restriction fragment length polymorphism analysis to clinical medicine, a clearer picture should emerge in the near future.

Lymphoproliferative disorders different from the original disease usually develop within a few months to one year after transplantation. Histology revealed pleomorphic B cell lymphoma to be most frequent with immunological evidence of initial polyclonal activation finally leading to monoclonal proliferation. However, other histologies have been observed as well. In most instances these lymphomas developed in cells of donor origin and in many cases Epstein-Barr virus genomic sequences could be identified in the cells.

The development of these lymphoproliferative disorders appears to be more frequent in patients given very aggressive immunosuppressive therapy, especially for the treatment of GVHD. Agents used include antithymocyte globulin, monoclonal antibodies, and cyclosporine. Lymphoproliferative disorders have also been observed in patients given marrow that had been depleted of T cells in vitro (using monoclonal antibodies and complement), and seem to be particularly frequent in patients given HLA nonidentical T cell dpeleted marrow. It has been postulated that the removal of T cells might result in a lack of regulation or in dysregulation of B lymphocytes. Present experience suggests that a more judicious use of immunosuppressive agents and a reduction in dose wherever possible may reduce the probability of such a malignancy developing.

Solid tumors were usually observed with a greater delay after transplantation, with intervals to occurrence ranging from 1 to approximately 14 years after transplantation. These malignancies have included glioblastoma multiform, adenocarcinomas, squamous cell carcinomas, basal cell carcinoma, malignant melanoma, and sarcomas. Data available to date suggest that for this group of patients irradiation may indeed be an etiologic factor. Superimposed may be an effect of chronic GVHD, an expression of continued (autoimmune) antigenic stimulation, and the treatment of GVHD with steroids or cytotoxic agents.

Only an occasional new leukemia in host cells has been observed. The etiology is not clear but may be similar to that of solid tumors.

Although the occurrence of secondary malignancies is of concern, several factors should be considered: first, most of these patients were initially treated for a potentially fatal illness, and without the use of marrow transplantation would have been expected to die within weeks or months. Second, malignant neoplasms have also been observed in nontransplant patients receiving chemotherapy only, or irradiation and chemotherapy without marrow transplantation. Third, it is conceivable that the development of a second neoplasm is favored by an underlying genetic defect, which had already led to the development of the initial hematologic malignancy. Regardless of the etiology, however, the overall incidence to date appears to be low (approximately 1%). Further follow-up studies are needed before a more definitive assessment of this problem can be made.

References

Boyd CN, Ramberg RC, Thomas ED (1982) The incidence of recurrence of leukemia in donor cells after allogeneic bone marrow transplantation. Leukemia Research 6: 833

Deeg HJ, Sanders J, Martin P, Fefer A, Neiman P, Singer J, Storb R, Thomas ED (1984) Secondary malignancies after marrow transplantation. Exp Hematol 12: 660

Fialkow PJ, Thomas ED, Bryant JI, Neiman PE (1971) Leukaemic transformation of engrafted human marrow cells in vivo. The Lancet I: 251

Marmont A, Frassoni F, Bacigalupo A, Podesta M, Piaggio G, Van Lint MT, Caimo A, de Filippi S (1984) Recurrence of Ph'-positive leukemia in donor cells after marrow transplantation for chronic granulocytic leukemia. 310: 903

Martin PJ, Shulman HM, Schubach WH, Hansen JA, Fefer A, Miller G, Thomas ED (1984) Fatal Epstein-Barr-virus-associated proliferation of donor B cells after treatment of acute graft-versus-host disease with a murine anti-T-cell antibody. Annals of Int Med 101: 310

Minden MD, Messner HA, Belch A (1985) Origin of leukemic relapse after bone marrow transplantation detected by restriction fragment length polymorphism. J Clin Invest 75: 91

Schubach WH, Miller G, Thomas ED (1985) Epstein-Barr virus genomes are restricted to secondary neoplastic cells following bone marrow transplantation. Blood 65: 535

Shapiro RS, Pietryga D, Blazar BR, Greenberg J, McClain K, Kersey K, Ramsay NKC, Filipovich AH (1987) B cell lymphoproliferative disorders following bone marrow transplantation. Progress in Bone Marrow Transplantation R. P. Gale and R. Champlin (eds.) Alan R. Liss, Inc., New York, pp. 647

Witherspoon RP, Schubach W, Neiman P, Martin P, Thomas ED (1985) Donor cell leukemia developing six years after marrow grafting for acute leukemia. Blood 65: 1172

7. Long-Term Adjustments

Although marrow transplantation is now being carried out at several hundred centers world wide, an assessment of long-term adjustment post transplant is still preliminary. Based on the above discussions, it should be clear that long-term adjustment will depend strongly upon the patient's underlying disease, the conditioning regimen used in preparation for marrow transplantation, and the patient's age and social status at the time of transplantation. Patients with non-malignant diseases prepared for marrow transplantation by chemotherapy alone, in particular regimens involving only the use of cyclophosphamide, clearly do very well, return to work promptly, are productive, grow and develop normally, are in many instances fertile, andl lead essentially normal lives unless severe chronic GVHD develops. If patients suffer from a malignancy and are prepared with more aggressive conditioning, especially the use of total body irradiation, more severe delayed effects are expected. Children of both sexes show a retardation of growth, and presumably never reach their normal height. Furthermore, they are likely to have abnormal sexual development, and in most instances will be sterile. These are important factors to consider, particularly since these problems may become relevant in patients only many years after transplantation when the original trauma is almost forgotten, and is not sufficient for an explanation for problems encountered at a later point in time. This requires very sensitive and close psychological guidance. It may affect schooling of young patients, and the professional careers of adult patients who occasionally may choose a career change.

Also, many patients, possibly more male than female, will encounter problems in their sexual life, frequently in the form of impotence. All available data suggest that this is usually a psychological, rather than a somatic problem. However, it requires attention and time on the part of the physician, and a diligent handling of the relevant questions in meetings with the patient alone, as well as in the company of the spouse. Despite all efforts, however, it appears that the stress on marital relationships is severe as judged by the number of separations or divorces in the course of, or following, marrow transplantation. It is likely that these problems are not only related to the post transplantation course but were affected as well by the diagnosis of the patient's original disease, the emotional, social, and financial stresses associated with it, the disruption of professional and personal lives, and the questionable outlook associated with such a disease even in view of the improving results with marrow transplantation.

Data on the psychological and intellectual development of children are only gradually becoming available. The first impression is that these children behave similarly to children with leukemia who have been given aggressive chemoradiotherapy. That is, although some learning disabilities have been encountered, in general these children are able to complete their education in normal schools.

VI. Future Developments

Bone marrow transplantation is a complex procedure. However, the basic purpose is that of transfering normally functioning lymphohemopoietic stem cells for lymphohemopoietic reconstitution and to supply cells with normal genetic information central to metabolic pathways in the recipient organism. Consequently, the future of marrow transplantation will depend upon improving the efficiency and efficacy of these functions. Quite likely the next generation of marrow transplantation phenomenologically will be quite different from the procedures used at the present time. The most important problems still to be mastered are those of recurrence of the underlying disease, prevention of GVHD without jeopardizing engraftment, prevention of infection, and prevention of delayed adverse effects.

Preventing recurrence of leukemia, lymphoma, or other malignancies will require a more effective eradication of clonogenic tumor cells than is possible at present. Currently employed regimens are generally already at maximum tolerated intensity. This is true for both chemotherapeutic and irradiation approaches. It is possible that combinations of different agents similar to combined modality treatment of lymphohemopoietic malignancies or solid tumors will have improved efficacy in eradicating malignant cells. Assuming that non-marrow toxicity is not prohibitive, marrow infusion used as a rescue procedure should then result in cure of most patients. However, at the present time quick progress in this field appears unlikely. What other options remain? Experimental studies indicate that coupling of radioisotopes to monoclonal antibodies directed at tumor cells might allow for in situ delivery of highdose radiation without unacceptable damage to organs other than the lymphohemopoietic system. A sufficiently rapid radioactive decay, so as to limit the time period of impaired marrow function prior to marrow infusion, would allow for successful application of this method. It may also be possible to couple immunotoxins such as ricin chain A to monoclonal antibodies for in vivo/ex vivo treatment of remaining tumor cells.

The long described graft-vs-leukemia effect still remains intriguing, although clinical studies attempting to take advantage of such an effect to reduce the probability of leukemic relapse and improve survival have been less than convincing. If data obtained in murine systems can be extrapolated, it should be possible to separate a graft-vs-leukemia effect from a graft-vs-host effect which in turn would allow for reduced recurrence rates without putting the patient at risk of dying from GVHD associated problems. One might speculate that a modification of the approach that has become known as "lymphokine activated killer cells" could be applicable in marrow transplantation. It is of interest that a few cases of patients with chronic myelogenous leukemia have been reported who showed a transient cytogenetic relapse (in the form of Philadelphia chromosome positive cells) after transplantation. Subsequently, Philadelphia chromosome positive cells disappeared, and the patients have been followed and found to remain in remission. It is conceivable that the reappearance of these cells might have triggered a leukemia-reactive donor-derived cell clone, leading to the elimination of the leukemic cells.

Progress has been made in regards to the prevention of GVHD. Regimens using combinations of cyclosporine and methylprednisolone, or cyclosporine and methotrexate, have reduced the incidence of clinically relevant acute GVHD to approximately 20–30% of patients given HLA identical marrow grafts. The incidence of GVHD is still high in HLA non-identical marrow grafts. Also, chronic GVHD continues to be a problem. Furthermore, if a graft-vs-leukemia effect truly exists, one might speculate that profound immunosuppression in the form of a combination of drugs to decrease GVHD after transplantation might reduce such an effect, and result in increased probability of leukemic relapse. Conceivably, shortening the prophylactic immunosuppressive regimen might reduce that risk.

T-cell depletion of marrow by various techniques described above is now being used widely. It appears that successful depletion of T-cells by two or three logs, albeit successful in preventing GVHD, may also prevent successful (sustained) engraftment. It has been postulated that less complete depletion, i.e. leaving in place a certain number of T-lymphocytes, might facilitate engraftment and still allow for prevention of GVHD. This, however, is controversial. Alternatively, one could attempt more selective depletion, e.g. CD4 or CD8 positive T lymphocytes. In fact studies using this approach are underway but results to date are inconclusive or disappointing. Alternatively, complete T-cell depletion might be acceptable if other means are found to ensure engraftment. Several monoclonal antibodies directed at class I or II histocompatibility antigens, or radioresistant cells, have been used in murine and canine models, and an antibody directed at the human lymphocyte function antigen (LFA) 1 has been used successfully in facilitating engraftment, even of histoincompatible marrow. Finally, exciting data obtained in murine models show that mice transplanted with a combination of T-cell depleted autologous marrow and unmanipulated histoincompatible allogeneic marrow not only achieved engraftment but also failed to develop GVHD. Similar studies are currently underway in larger animals and in a pilot study in man (A. Gratwohl, personal communication). If successful, this approach will be attractive for more extensive clinical trials.

Another approach to the prevention of GVHD is the use of autologous marrow. In recent years, autologous marrow transplants have been carried out with increasing frequency and with good success rates for indications such as non-Hodgkin's lymphomas or acute non-lymphoblastic leukemias. A major problem, however, is the recurrence of the underlying disease. It is not clear whether this is due to proliferation of clonogenic cells surviving the conditioning regimen in the patient or tumor cells present in the marrow and re-infused following conditioning. Although a contribution by re-infused cells is possible, the high recurrence rate in certain patient groups even with allogeneic marrow transplantation suggests that the most important problem is that of relative inefficacy of the conditioning regimen. In agreement with this concept some investigators point out that there is no significant difference in relapse rate between patients given autologous purged or unpurged marrow. In any event, as far as eradication of tumor cells in the patient is concerned, approaches similar to those being tried for allogeneic transplants might be useful. In regards to marrow manipulation, recent experimental data suggest that approaches other than conventional purging might be possible. At least two groups have reported that in vitro culture of leukemic marrow (acute leukemia or Philadelphia chromosome positive chronic myelogenous leukemia) can lead to disappearance of malignant cells as suggested by disappearance of the respective chromosome abnormalities. Conceivably, cultured marrow could then be transplanted without the risk of re-introducing leukemia back into the patient. A first clinical study is currently under way.

As an alternative to autologous marrow, autologous peripheral blood could be used as a source of stem cells. Increased numbers of committed precursor cells can be obtained during a rebound phase following treatment of patients with cytotoxic agents. The feasibility of this approach has been shown in animals, and recent clinical data in small numbers of patients have shown successful hemopoietic reconstitution. Another advantage of this approach may be a lower contamination by tumor cells compared to bone marrow.

The next step would be direct enrichment, i.e. positive selection of actual stem cells. Experimental data in mice, dogs and monkeys indicate that such an approach is feasible for autologous transplantation. There is concern, however, that transplantation of purified stem cells may be problematic in the allogeneic setting due to problems with engraftment as described for T-cell depleted marrow (IV.3). Further experimental work is necessary. Conceivably, an accessory cell facilitating engraftment of stem cells could be infused concurrently. Alternatively, one could attempt to manipulate the stroma or microenvironment in the recipient in which stem cells are expected to settle. A lead in that direction may have been provided by the in vivo use of monoclonal antibodies in animals and man. We are currently developing a good unterstanding of the homing behaviour of lymphoid cell populations. However, very little is known about the homing of hemopoietic precursor cells. Once the responsible receptors have been recognized, manipulations could preferentially lodge stem cells in predetermined sites, such as the marrow cavity. The possibility that an accessory cell population participates in homing behaviour cannot be excluded.

For numerous indications, autologous stem cells clearly offer an alternative to allogeneic marrow transplantation. In certain diseases, for example severe aplastic anemia or congenital disorders, autologous stem cells, if available, would not be useful since the original disease would be reintroduced. However, only a limited number of patients have a suitable allogeneic donor as defined by presently accepted criteria. Consequently, it would be desirable to expand the donor pool by recruiting unrelated volunteer donors or by using cadaveric marrow. A national donor bank for volunteer marrow donors is currently being established in the United States and similar efforts are underway in the United Kingdom, Germany, and France. Logistically this task is not easy. Although several successful transplants from unrelated volunteer donors have been reported already, only a limited number of patients, specifically those with a commonly occurring HLA haplotype, are likely to find donors. Otherwise only HLA non-identical donors can be used and, hence, a major histocompatibility barrier has to be crossed with the associated increased risk of graft failure and GVHD. The same applies for cadaveric marrow. Although it is conceivable that large numbers of marrow cells could be obtained and enriched for stem cells, it is likely that cryopreservation will be necessary to store the marrow until use in an appropriate patient. These manipulations may lead to a loss of cells and to an increased risk of graft failure, both due to reduced cell viability and to resistance to engraftment (IV.3).

Another area of research that has reached the point of clinical application is that of hemopoietic growth factors. With the use of recombinant DNA technology large quantities of the various factors (e.g. Il 3, GM-CSF etc.) have become available and clinical pilot studies are underway. Conceivably, the use of these factors will accelerate hemopoietic reconstitution after autologous marrow transplantation and facilitate engraftment of T cell-depleted and stem cell-enriched fractions of allogeneic marrow. There is still concern, however, that growth factors may also stimulate leukemia cells, increasing the probability of leukemic relapse. Nonetheless, it is likely that individual factors or combinations thereof will be used successfully in leukemia, lymphoma or non-malignant hemopoietic disorders. The first clinical experience to be accrued is likely to be with autologous marrow transplantation for the treatment of solid tumors.

One of the most exciting areas at the present time is that of gene manipulation or gene transfer into stem cells. Although a large armamentarium of techniques and methodology is available, this approach is still plagued by problems with expression of the gene product after transfer to the recipient cells. However, once this hurdle is surmounted, the transfer of normal genetic information into autologous cells with defective or lacking information for the respective enzyme or molecule would be the treatment of choice for numerous congenital disorders such as immunedeficiencies, lysosomal storage diseases, and mucupolysaccharidoses. As it stands, however, manipulation of the recipient is necessary in order to generate a growth advantage for the cells transfected with the genetic material of interest. Hence, a more sophisticated transplantation technology allowing for those approaches needs to be developed.

Finally, considering the large numbers of patients that are given solid organ grafts such as kidney, liver, heart, heart/lung and pancreas, generally requiring indefinite immunosuppressive treatment with all the associated risks, it would be highly desirable to develop methods to provide an organ transplant recipient with an immune system that would accept the transplanted organ indefinitely without requiring continued immunosuppression. The transfer of marrow cells with selective immunocompetent cells tolerant to the transplant organ would be such an approach. Eventually this might even be feasible with xenogeneic grafts.

In summary, present and future work in the field of marrow transplantation will aim at more effective eradication of malignant cells, stem cell enrichment, improved allogeneic engraftment, abrogation of resistance to manipulated grafts and accelerated immunoreconstitution along with graft tolerance. Molecular biology techniques need to be developed to allow for consistent expression of transfected genes in stem cells, and together with actual transplant efforts, allow for preferential survival of the transfected cells in the recipient.

References

Badger CC, Krohn KA, Peterson AV, Shulman HM, Bernstein I (1985) Experimental radiotherapy of murine lymphoma with ^{131}I-labeled anti-Thy 1.1 monoclonal antibody. Cancer Res 45: 1536

Belmont JW, Tigges JH, Chang SMW, Smith KW, Kellems RE, Dick JE, Magli MC, Phillips RA, Bernstein A, Caskey CT (1986) Expression of human adenosine deaminase in murine haematopoietic progenitor cells following retroviral transfer. Nature 322: 385

Blume KG, Forman SJ, O'Donnell MR, Doroshow JH, Krance RA, Nademanee AP, Snyder DS, Schmidt GM, Fahey JL, Metter GE, Hill LR, Findley DO, Sniecinski IJ (1987) Total body irradiation and high-dose etoposide: A new preparatory regimen for bone marrow transplantation in patients with advanced hematologic malignancies. Blood 69: 1015

Buckner CD, Appelbaum FR, Clift RA, Doney K, Sanders J, Hill R, Thomas ED (1987) Autotransplants in leukemia: Do they work, how can we tell? Progress in Bone Marrow Transplantation RP Gale and R. Champlin (eds.) Alan R. Liss, Inc., New York p 711

Cheever MA, Greenberg PD, Fefer A (1984) Potential for specific cancer therapy with immune T lymphocytes. J Biol Response Modifiers 3: 113

Coloumbel L, Kalousek DK, Eaves CJ, Gupta CM, Eaves AC (1983) Longterm marrow culture reveals chromosomally normal hematopoietic progenitor cells in patients with Philadelphia chromosome positive chromic myelogenous leukemia. N Eng J Med 308: 1493

Ilstad ST and Sachs DH (1984) Reconstitution with syngeneic plus allogeneic or xenogeneic bone marrow leads to specific acceptance of allografts or xenografts. Nature 307: 168

Jalkanen S, Reichert RA, Gallatin WM, Bargartze RF, Weissmann IL, Butcher EC (1986) Homing receptors and the control of lymphocyte migration. Immunol Reviews 91: 39

Metcalf D (1986) The molecular biology and functions of the GM-CSFs. Blood 67: 257

Truitt RL, LeFever AV, Shih CC-Y (1987) Graft-versus-leukemia reactions: Experimental models and clinical trials. Progress in Bone Marrow Transplantation RP Gale and R Champlin (eds.) Alan R. Liss, Inc., New York, p 219

Reiffers J, Bernard P, David B, Vezon G, Sarrat A, Marit G, Moulinier J, Broustet A (1986) Successful autologous transplantation with peripheral blood hemopoietic cells in a patient with acute leukemia. Exp Hematol 14: 312

Wegmann TG, Rosovsky J, Carlson GA, Diener E, Drell DW (1980) Models for the production of stable hematopoietic chimerism across major histocompatibility barriers in adults. J Immunol 125: 1751

VII. Glossary

Allogeneic:	From a different individual of the same species.
Autologous (= autochthonous):	From the same individual; in marrow transplantation this means from the patient.
Bone marrow transplantation:	The intravenous infusion of marrow cells obtained by multiple aspirates from the bones (usually the posterior iliac crests) of the donor, into the recipient (patient, host). The relevant marrow cells (stem cells) find their way to the bone by a mechanism termed "homing" (via the nutritional arteries), settle in "niches" and begin to replicate and repopulate the patient's marrow cavities and blood.
Chimera:	An individual who hosts (indefinitely) cells of different genetic origin. In a marrow chimera, the donor-derived cells repopulate the patient's hemopoietic and immune system. For example if a transplant is carried out from a female donor into a male patient and the transplant is successful, the patient will have female lymphohemopoietic cells for the rest of his life.
Conditioning:	The preparation of the patient for marrow transplantation. Conditioning is aimed at eradicating the patient's own cells (malignant cells of the disease for which treatment is being given, and immuno-competent cells of the patient's immune system) to allow for engraftment of donor cells. Conditioning may include the use of gamma irradiation, cytotoxic and immunosuppressive drugs, monoclonal or polyclonal antibodies, and in the near future possible radioisotopes and immunotoxins.
Donor:	The individual from whom the marrow cells (or blood cells used for transfusions) are obtained.

Engraftment:	About 2–3 weeks after infusion of bone marrow, granulocytes (in the case of allogeneic transplantation of donor origin) appear in the peripheral blood indicating that donor cells have begun to replicate, i.e. the transplant has engrafted. Engraftment can also be demonstrated by bone marrow biopsy which shows granulocyte, red blood cell, and platelet precursors usually around day 14.
Graft-versus-host disease (GVHD):	Presumably all transplants other than autologous or syngeneic result in a graft-versus-host reaction, i.e. an interaction between donor-derived and host cells. If a state of tolerance develops, there may be no manifestations of this interaction. In many instances, however, this interaction may result in tissue damage especially to skin, intestinal tract and liver, and lead to clinical dysfunction of those organs, termed GVHD. This reaction is triggered by donor-derived T cells.
HLA:	Abbreviation for "Human Leukocyte Antigens". These antigens were found originally on leukocytes, especially lymphocytes, but some of them (HLA class I antigens) are expressed widely and possibly on all nucleated cells. The genetic information that is responsible for the expression of these antigens is located on the short arm of chromosome 6 in a region called the major histocompatibility complex. Within this complex, dependent upon structure and function, three clases (I, II and III) of antigens are distinguished. Class I antigens are defined biochemically as dimers of a glycoprotein of 45 Kd molecular weight, linked noncovalently to beta 2-microglobulin. Class II antigens (Ia-like antigens) are defined biochemically as glycoprotein dimers of approximately 29 and 34 Kd molecular weight respectively. These HLA antigens play a central role in the interaction of immunocompetent cells, and in the interaction between donor and host cells. They are also responsible for mutual recognition of cells in mixed leukocyte culture. Class III antigens represent complement components.
Host:	The recipient of a transplant (of marrow or a solid organ) i.e. the patient.
Host-versus-graft reaction:	A function of host cells with a detrimental effect on donor cells. If the host-versus-graft reaction is stronger than the graft-versus-host reaction, it will result in rejection (or non-acceptance) of the graft, i.e. the graft fails (does not take).

Mismatch:	If host and donor HLA type (A, B, D/DR) are not genotypically identical, a mismatch situation exists. This includes the rare case of phenotypic identity, where the various antigens appear to be the same in donor and host but family studies show that they are derived from a different genetic background. If one, two or three antigens are phenotypically different we refer to a one, two or three antigen (one haplotype) mismatch.
Mixed Lymphocyte Culture (MLC):	Lymphocytes of patient and donor are co-cultured for 6 days in tissue culture plates. Usually one cell population is inactivated by irradiation or mitomycin. If lymphocytes of patient and donor differ at the HLA D/DR region, the non-inactivated population will proliferate. The amount of proliferation, measured by thymidine incorporation, can be used as a relative measure of histoincompatibility between donor and patient.
Non-HLA antigens:	Histocompatibility antigens other than HLA, also called minor antigens, encoded for by genes outside the major histocompatibility complex and often on different chromosomes. In man these antigens are poorly defined.
Syngeneic:	From a different but genetically identical individual, i.e. from a monozygotic twin.
Xenogeneic:	From an individual of a different species.

SPRINGER NATURE

GPSR Compliance

The European Union's (EU) General Product Safety Regulation (GPSR) is a set of rules that requires consumer products to be safe and our obligations to ensure this.

If you have any concerns about our products, you can contact us on ProductSafety@springernature.com

In case Publisher is established outside the EU, the EU authorized representative is:

Springer Nature Customer Service Center GmbH
Europaplatz 3
69115 Heidelberg, Germany

FSC
www.fsc.org
MIX
Papier | Fördert gute Waldnutzung
FSC® C083411

Kolibri 360 GmbH
Ferdinand-Jühlke-Straße 7
99095 Erfurt, Deutschland
produktsicherheit@kolibri360.de